PRACTICAL ASTIGMATISM
Planning and Analysis

PRACTICAL ASTIGMATISM
Planning and Analysis

**NOEL ALPINS, AM, MB, BS, DO (MELB),
FRANZCO, FRACS, FRCOPHTH, FACS**
MEDICAL DIRECTOR
NEWVISION CLINICS
CLINICAL SENIOR LECTURER
DEPARTMENT OF OPHTHALMOLOGY
MELBOURNE UNIVERSITY
VICTORIA, AUSTRALIA

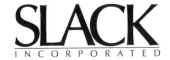

www.Healio.com/books

ISBN: 978-1-61711-995-8

The procedures and practices described in this publication should be implemented in a manner consistent with the professional standards set for the circumstances that apply in each specific situation. Every effort has been made to confirm the accuracy of the information presented and to correctly relate generally accepted practices. The authors, editors, and publisher cannot accept responsibility for errors or exclusions or for the outcome of the material presented herein. There is no expressed or implied warranty of this book or information imparted by it. Care has been taken to ensure that drug selection and dosages are in accordance with currently accepted/recommended practice. Off-label uses of drugs may be discussed. Due to continuing research, changes in government policy and regulations, and various effects of drug reactions and interactions, it is recommended that the reader carefully review all materials and literature provided for each drug, especially those that are new or not frequently used. Some drugs or devices in this publication have clearance for use in a restricted research setting by the Food and Drug and Administration or FDA. Each professional should determine the FDA status of any drug or device prior to use in their practice.

Any review or mention of specific companies or products is not intended as an endorsement by the author or publisher.

SLACK Incorporated uses a review process to evaluate submitted material. Prior to publication, educators or clinicians provide important feedback on the content that we publish. We welcome feedback on this work.

Published by: SLACK Incorporated
                    6900 Grove Road
                    Thorofare, NJ 08086 USA
                    Telephone: 856-848-1000
                    Fax: 856-848-6091
                    www.Healio.com/books

Contact SLACK Incorporated for more information about other books in this field or about the availability of our books from distributors outside the United States.

Library of Congress Cataloging-in-Publication Data

Names: Alpins, Noel, author.
Title: Practical astigmatism : planning and analysis / Noel Alpins.
Description: Thorofare, NJ : Slack Incorporated, [2018] | Includes
  bibliographical references and index.
Identifiers: LCCN 2017031601| ISBN 9781617119958 (hardback) | ISBN
  9781630915278 (epub) | ISBN 9781630915285 (web)
Subjects: | MESH: Astigmatism--surgery
Classification: LCC RE932 | NLM WW 310 | DDC 617.7/19059--dc23 LC record available at
https://lccn.loc.gov/2017031601

Printed in the United States of America.

Last digit is print number: 10   9   8   7   6   5   4   3   2   1

DEDICATION

This book is dedicated to my wife, Sylvia. Her love and encouragement were always there even when the pursuit of the "Alpins Method" had me distracted from giving her all the attention she deserved. Many times, I was away when I might have been home, and many other times, we traveled to far-away places together, which might not have happened if the epiphany of 1992 had not put us on a path of discovery. Her patience under my cloud of distraction has been the foundation for my enthusiasm. Sylvia was there every minute of every day. At one point, around the year 2000, she asked me, "When will all this be over?" This was a question, I must admit, that had been reverberating with some insistence around the depths of my own psyche. However, the answer, as we were to discover, was that it's over when it's over. This enthusiasm, and my appreciation for her, have only made us closer.

Through the 1990s and into the new century, I traveled extensively, sometimes with my family, but often without Sylvia or our three daughters, Fiona, Vanessa, and Martine, who have gone on to successful, satisfying lives in their own right, that of which Sylvia and I are justly proud. If I have regrets, they revolve around those many hours where my path took me away from a loving home. I can only hope that, in the end, it was worth it to all involved. This book is for you. As for me, most of the answers might now have been achieved.

CONTENTS

ACKNOWLEDGMENTS

As one can imagine, the actual mechanical preparation of a book is a team effort. I'd like to especially thank George Stamatelatos, BScOptom, my frequent coauthor and invaluable assistant at my practice in Melbourne, Australia, and many others at my practice who helped administratively. Editorially, I extend my appreciation to Tony Schiavo, an editor at SLACK Incorporated, a Wyanoke Group company; April Billick, who coordinated the design of the cover; and Keith Croes, a freelance editor and former employee of *Ocular Surgery News* who has gone on to work in a variety of medical specialties. The worldwide task of compiling and, often, redrawing of figures was effectively overseen by Martha Slawek. Thank you to James Ong for his brilliant mathematical mind and contribution of the astigmatism analyses in Chapter 23. My special thanks to Peter Slack, of SLACK Incorporated, who was instrumental in getting the project started from its earliest days.

I'd also like to acknowledge all who have helped me on this journey, many of whom I've tried to identify and to thank as appropriately within these pages. Nothing of any substance is accomplished in science or within a medical specialty without the input of many, and in my case, there are a significant number who have names I never knew. To the doctors who approached me at different meetings throughout the world, with a look of understanding in their eyes, and acknowledged, "I think I get it"; to the unnamed editors, attorneys, friends, and acquaintances with good ideas that perhaps later affected my approaches (or bent the trajectory of the arrow), this book testifies to your individual contributions. I thank you all with all my heart.

ABOUT THE AUTHOR

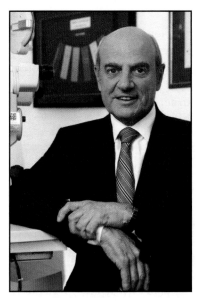

Dr. Alpins pioneered small-incision cataract surgery in Victoria, Australia, in 1987 and then became a founder and current member of the Excimer Laser & Research Group. He has specialized in cataract and refractive surgery since founding NewVision Clinics in Melbourne, Australia, in 1996. He speaks widely on surgical techniques at national and international meetings and has been a keynote speaker and chair on many occasions.

Dr. Alpins serves on the Royal Australian and New Zealand College of Ophthalmologists (RANZCO) program committee, and has served as chair for the invited speakers subcommittee since 2008. In 2010, he was the invited Council Lecturer at the RANZCO annual scientific meeting in Adelaide, South Australia, which was established to honor Fellows engaged in original work.

In addition to his many writings and lectures, he continues to investigate the vector analytic approach to astigmatism analysis that he pioneered (the Alpins Method). He is involved in ongoing clinical research in this area. He is also an international council member of the International Society of Refractive Surgery (ISRS) of the American Academy of Ophthalmology (AAO).

Dr. Alpins is on the editorial board of a number of publications, including the *Journal of Cataract & Refractive Surgery* (official journal of the American Society of Cataract and Refractive Surgery and the European Society of Cataract and Refractive Surgeons), the *Journal of Refractive Surgery* (a publication of the International Society of Refractive Surgery affiliated with the American Academy of Ophthalmology), *Ocular Surgery News, EuroTimes,* and others. He has contributed over 150 articles in peer-reviewed journals and ophthalmic periodicals as well as more than 20 book chapters. In 2015, he received the Certificate for Outstanding Contribution in Reviewing, awarded by Elsevier.

Dr. Alpins received the 2012 ISRS/AAO Lans Distinguished Award in Chicago, and in 2014 he received the ISRS Lifetime Achievement Award. Dr. Alpins is on the international advisory board for refractive surgery in China.

In January 2017, Dr. Alpins was awarded Member in the General Division of the Order of Australia for "significant service to ophthalmology, particularly to the development of innovative refractive surgery techniques, and to professional associations." The Order of Australia was established in 1975 by letters patent of Elizabeth II, Queen of Australia, and countersigned by Prime Minister Gough Whitlam. Around 500 prominent Australians receive the award annually. Dr. Alpins is also regularly appointed as an ambassador for the state of Victoria in the government's annual Australia Day.

Dr. Alpins is the 2017 RANZCO "Norman McAlister Gregg Lecturer" for 2017. The Gregg Lecture was established in 1958 by the Council of the Ophthalmological Society of Australia in recognition of the outstanding contribution made to ophthalmology by Sir Norman Gregg.

Dr. Alpins and his wife, Sylvia, have three daughters: Fiona, Vanessa, and Martine. When Dr. Alpins is not practicing ophthalmology, he enjoys playing golf, skiing, going to live entertainment, and spending time with Sylvia, his daughters, and grandchildren.

His training is summarized below:

- Medical degree (MB, BS): University of Melbourne, 1970
- Diploma of Ophthalmology: University of Melbourne, 1977
- Residency: Alfred Hospital, Australia, 1971-1972
- Fellowships and certifications: Ophthalmology Registrar, Royal Victoria Eye & Ear Hospital, Australia, 1974-77; Fellow, RANZCO, 1978; Fellow, Royal Australasian College of Surgeons, 1978; Fellow, American College of Surgeons, 1985; Fellow, Royal College of Ophthalmologists (UK), 1989; Fellow, American Board of Eye Surgery, 2005; Honorary Senior Lecturer, Melbourne University Department of Ophthalmology, 2013.
- Memberships: International Intra-Ocular Implant Club; American Society of Cataract and Refractive Surgery; European Society of Cataract and Refractive Surgeons; International Society of Refractive Surgery; American Academy of Ophthalmology; and the Australian Medical Association.

PREFACE

I gave my first talk on astigmatism in 1986 at an Australian college meeting, the Royal Australian and New Zealand College of Ophthalmologists (RANZCO) in Melbourne, Australia. I discussed what I called "dynamic vector analysis," a process I named after a long period of Friday-morning appointments spent removing sutures after cataract extraction in a way to minimize or rotate astigmatism. I stopped performing extracapsular cataract extraction in 1987, primarily because both the surgery and the follow-up consumed so much time.

As it turned out, I was the first ophthalmologist to adopt phacoemulsification in Melbourne. I learned it primarily from the Sinskey course in Los Angeles. I also watched a lot of videos, including ones by Howard Gimbel. In 1986, I met Howard "Under the Banyan Tree" at the Royal Hawaiian Eye Meeting (RHEM), and his mentorship helped my transition to phacoemulsification. Howard's influence was inspirational for the next decade.

In January 1987 at RHEM, I met Spencer Thornton. I had started performing radial keratotomy (RK) in 1985; soon after meeting Dr. Thornton, he visited me in Australia and I adopted astigmatic keratotomy (AK) in the manner he described (see Chapter 2). The AK incisions became arcuate a couple years later. Jaffe and Clayman had previously discussed pre- and postoperative vectors,[1] with the hypotenuse of the triangle being the surgical induced astigmatism vector (SIA); I believe I adequately credited these and other pioneers in my work to come.

In 1992, ViSX (Johnson & Johnson) introduced an elliptical zone for astigmatic ablative corrections and a new paradigm began. It wasn't long before I realized that corneal analysis in contrast to refractive analysis required a nonzero target. It took me 3 years (1993 through 1996) to figure out all the relationships and indices involved. I did not fully adopt laser in situ keratomileusis (LASIK) until 1997. For me, the breakthrough was related to computerization, analysis, and planning.

To some, these relationships seemed apparent and I often heard others intone, "That was easy." I must be a little dense, as it took me 3 years to make the full vectorial and operative associations inherent in the Alpins Method. In the back of my mind, I also knew that it can take up to 20 years for a fundamental change to take effect in any medical specialty.

My first publication on the Alpins Method dates to 1993,[2] but it was not until 2006 that an "official" attempt was made to co-opt my approach.[3] The details and ramifications of this are fully described elsewhere in this book.

Suffice it to say that time could have been spent more productively if some adept colleagues and I had not devoted our resources to resolving what I consider, for the most part, to be inane and obvious terminology errors. It is unfortunate, but there is a happy ending. All of our major journals now support the use of the Alpins Method in designing and reporting studies that include astigmatism analysis.[3-8]

References

1. Jaffe NS, Clayman HM. The pathophysiology of corneal astigmatism after cataract extraction. *Transactions of the American Academy of Ophthalmology and Otolaryngology.* Rochester, MN: 1975:OP-615-OP-630.

2. Alpins NA. A new method of analyzing vectors for changes in astigmatism. *J Cataract Refract Surg.* 1993;19(4):524-533.

3. Eydelman MB, Drum B, Holladay J, et al. Standardized analyses of correction of astigmatism by laser systems that reshape the cornea. *J Refract Surg.* 2006;22(1):81-95.

4. Author Information Pack. Elsevier Web site. https://www.elsevier.com/wps/find/journaldescription. cws_home/620418?generatepdf=true. Accessed January 19, 2016.

5. Information for Authors. Journal of Cataract & Refractive Surgery Web site. http://www.jcrsjournal. org/content/authorinfo#info. Accessed September 1, 2016.

6. Reinstein DZ, Archer TJ, Randleman JB. JRS standard for reporting astigmatism outcomes of refractive surgery [editorial]. *J Refract Surg.* 2014;30(10):654-659.

7. Reinstein DZ, Archer TJ, Srinivasan S, et al. Standard for reporting refractive outcomes of intraocular lens-based refractive surgery. *J Refract Surg.* 2017;33(4):218-222.

8. Reinstein DZ, Archer TJ, Srinivasan S, et al. Standard for reporting refractive outcomes of intraocula lens-based refractive surgery. *J Refract Surg.* 2017;43(4):435-439.

FOREWORD

EXPANDED BOUNDARIES IN A NEW ERA

Ophthalmic surgery is entering an exciting new era, with the goals for a better, optical result. The technology is rapidly changing, our boundaries are expanding, and today, our patients can expect to achieve excellent visual results. This book reveals the discoveries that have made possible these remarkable breakthroughs.

Over the past quarter century, great advances have been made in restoring vision to optical levels better than any previously available. The goal 4 or 5 decades ago was to restore vision after cataract removal without resorting to thick cataract spectacles; today, with astigmatism-correcting surgery, we are able to provide clarity of vision unequaled even by the natural lens and "nonastigmatic" optical systems.

In correcting astigmatism, patients are much more interested in their visual outcome than the technology used, and so the surgeon needs to make decisions that will meet patients' needs without confusing them with choices that only a scientist can understand. They are more interested in what you tell them about how they will be able to see.

The method of astigmatism analysis explained in this book recognizes the need to define a specific goal, thus, allowing the surgeon to obtain precise, separate measures of the magnitude and the angle of surgical error. From this, the surgeon can evaluate what surgery may be required to achieve the preoperative goal. An index that measures surgical success is adjusted for the level of preoperative astigmatism.

The resulting data allow statistical comparison of multiple surgical methods and techniques, and help resolve cases where spectacle and corneal astigmatism do not coincide.

The Alpins Method addresses astigmatism using vector analysis, a method introduced by Dr. Noel Alpins in the 1990s (and others in various ways) and refined over the decades since. In this book, Dr. Alpins reveals a new understanding of coupling and the effect of position, depth, and length of corneal incisions. He goes into the history of approaches to astigmatism correction with thoroughness not often seen in textbooks. The reader will see the value of vector analysis in treating all types of astigmatism, both developmental and iatrogenic.

In explaining vectors, Dr. Alpins goes into the mathematics of magnitude and direction in easily understandable ways, pointing out that vector analysis involves the application of values from topographers, keratometers, wavefront aberrometers, autorefractors, etc. The result of this analysis can make astigmatism surgery more precise and patient-pleasing.

As the technology of astigmatism correction continues to evolve and improve, it is reassuring to see this classic work on the Alpins Method presented to the profession. As Dr. Alpins shows, it is clear that the technology should be determined for the eye, not the eye for the technology. There is no one-size-fits-all method.

Incision Versus Ablation

This book explains the differences between incisional and ablative approaches to astigmatism correction and why the Alpins Method is a major advance. He discusses the various approaches to surgery and credits the developers of each method.

It is clear that the Alpins Method of astigmatism analysis is a major advance in cataract and corneal transplant surgery. His definition of terms (ORA, TIA, SIA, DV, etc) makes the work valuable to the new or experienced surgeon. Although his initial publication of the Alpins Method was in 1993, it has been only over the past few years that his terminology, and almost every other aspect of his work, has been embraced as the standard for astigmatism reporting going forward. This standard holds now for our major journals, the *Journal of Cataract & Refractive Surgery*, the *Journal of Refractive Surgery*, and *Ophthalmology*. The *Journal of Cataract & Refractive Surgery* is the official publication of the American Society of Cataract and Refractive Surgery (ASCRS). The *Journal of Refractive Surgery* is the official publication of the International Society of Refractive Surgery, a sister organization to the American Academy of Ophthalmology, whose official publication is *Ophthalmology*.

The Chapters Ahead of You

This book deals with noncorneal astigmatism (ocular residual astigmatism, or ORA) in an understandable and practical way. As you will find ahead, the existence of ORA provided early inspiration and motivation for the eventual completion of what has come to be known as the "Alpins Method."

Correct terminology is important and is addressed frequently in the book, and in a separate section at the end, as are the concepts of flattening, steepening, and rotation of astigmatism, which have particular relevance in cataract incisional surgery and addressed in Chapter 8.

Dr. Alpins discusses the advances brought about by toric intraocular lenses (IOLs) as well as the sometimes necessary correction of resultant astigmatism with these lenses. The new concepts of corneal topographic astigmatism (CorT) anterior and CorT total—which I believe have the potential of also becoming standard approaches in the future to replace the less reliable simulated keratometry (SimK)—are described in detail.

The Alpins Method employs important ideas such as the Vector Planning® approach and the concept of "less is more" when it comes to astigmatism in refractive laser surgery; benefits that may lead to an improved level of patient satisfaction.

The "hemidivisional solution" and "topographic disparity," basically represent the application of the Alpins Method to people with irregular astigmatism, a significant population in a refractive surgical practice. Again, I believe these concepts comprise a new standard, applicable to quantifying corneal irregularity relevant to all topographers and introduced and available through the iASSORT® software program.

Every major contribution, in every major area of human endeavor—from medical-scientific disciplines to social and political movements—has detractors or opponents or others who simply believe they have "a better idea." The Alpins Method is no exception. I have never read a "behind-the-scenes" look in a medical specialty textbook as you'll find here (Chapters 18 and 20).

In conclusion—and importantly—this work is thoroughly referenced and illustrated, and maintains a refreshing, and sometimes humorous style, as if you were having a conversation with Dr. Alpins on the subject. It is a tribute to him, and offers a unique "insightful" flavor I find eminently digestible. I recommend it to all practicing ophthalmologists and ophthalmologists in training.

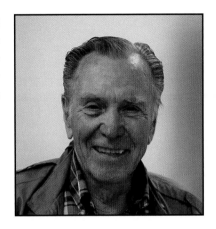

Spencer P. Thornton, MD, FACS
Clinical Professor of Ophthalmology
Department of Ophthalmology
University of Tennessee Health Science Center
Memphis, Tennessee

FOREWORD

THE ALPINS METHOD IS THE FOUNDATION FOR THE TERMINOLOGY OF ASTIGMATISM REPORTING

Astigmatism, and the analysis of astigmatism in particular, is one of the most challenging areas of refractive surgery for many ophthalmologists due to the relative complexity of the mathematics required. Noel Alpins has made formalizing the analysis of astigmatism in refractive surgery his life's work, as summarized in this book, for which we all owe him a great debt. While the basic concepts of using vectors to describe astigmatism had been set down many years earlier, Noel's work constructed a complete methodology to apply to any surgical situation, built around the central concept of the non-zero target, and the consideration of both refractive and corneal astigmatism. Over the years, a number of other methods for analyzing astigmatic outcomes have been described, and while each serves its purpose, it has become widely agreed that the Alpins Method provides the best, all-around interpretation.

Along the way, Noel described and defined the range of parameters required for his method. Having been keenly aware of his work and presence on the podium, my real introduction to Noel came in 2009 through the topic of terminology following the publication of the editorial I co-authored with George Waring III that updated the Standard Graphs for Refractive Surgery for the *Journal of Refractive Surgery*.[1] But to tell the full story, we need to rewind back to 2006 and to the confusion surrounding astigmatism terminology.

In 2006, an attempt to address the question of a minimum standard format for reporting astigmatic outcomes was proposed by the Astigmatism Project Group of the American National Standards Institute (ANSI), led by Malvina Eydelman, director for the Division of Ophthalmic and Ear, Nose & Throat Devices at the United States Food and Drug Administration (FDA). The final report was subsequently published in the *Journal of Refractive Surgery*[2]; however, the article was not subject to peer-review on the basis that the article was a completed formal document from ANSI and that the content was the final report from the project's group.[3] The majority of the astigmatism analysis methods described in the ANSI article[2] were based on the Alpins Method[4-6]; however the terminology was renamed (possibly because the committee thought that the new terms might be better descriptors).

In response to the publication of this report, Noel submitted a letter to the editor that raised this issue, and the concern that changing the terminology would create confusion.[7] Further support for the Alpins Method and use of the original terminology was published later that year in an editorial by Koch.[8] Unfortunately, the damage was done and the analysis and terminology described in the ANSI report[2] has since been used in numerous papers,[9-11] based on the authority associated with the connection to the FDA and publication in the *Journal of Refractive Surgery*. As has been elegantly described in an editorial by Dupps,[12] it is common for authors to be more aware of recent publications, so there is always a risk that a primary source can get lost during the evolutionary citation process if some authors start referencing more recent publications only. In the editorial, Dupps[12] addresses the question of the Alpins Method as a specific example:

Finally omission of key references or attribution of work to a secondary reference rather than a primary source can distort the field by re-mapping key contribution inaccurately. This challenging issue, a recently noted example of which is Alpins'[6] under-acknowledged vector approach to analyzing surgically induced astigmatism can be addressed through errata and correspondences;[8] but once in the literature, such errors are prone to propagation. Errors of omission or inaccurate attribution also occur when review articles are used in lieu of primary sources.

It is an easy mistake to make, which is exactly what we did when publishing our astigmatic results of topography-guided treatments in eyes with irregular astigmatism.[13] As the ANSI report[2] had been published in the *Journal of Refractive Surgery*, we (mis) interpreted this as being the journal's standard and followed it to the letter. It never occurred to us to refer back to the original source for the correct terminology, nor were we aware of Noel's letter to the editor. However, our biggest mistake was to later refer to the article as "a standard for reporting cylinder vector analysis," within the 2009 *Journal of Refractive Surgery* editorial that updated the Standard Graphs for Reporting Refractive Surgery.[1]

I was quickly contacted by Noel after this editorial was published and he explained the full history of the ANSI report and pointed out how the terminology had been renamed. Over the next years, together with first George Waring III, and then Brad Randleman, we set about formally resolving the confusion over terminology. This was finally achieved in our editorial published in 2014 that expanded the Standard Graphs for Reporting Refractive Surgery to include vector analysis of refractive cylinder.[14] The relevant section on terminology is worth quoting in full:

> Our position at the Journal is that all future reports of astigmatism should adhere to the original terminology as described by Alpins.[4-6] There are three reasons for this, and the guiding principle is clarity in communication above all else. The Alpins terminology has been in use for more than 20 years and had been in use for 13 years prior to the ANSI article,[2] and so had already become widely used in the field within hundreds of publications. Because there is no added clarity in using the new terminology, there is no benefit to alternative strategies for describing the same thing; different terminology can only cause unnecessary confusion to readers. We further agree with the basic principle of acknowledging primary source material, as has been recently highlighted by Dupps.[12] It is common for authors to be more aware of recent publications, so there is always a risk that a primary source can get lost during the evolutionary citation process if some authors start referencing the more recent publication only. It is an easy mistake to make; we have been guilty of doing exactly this, for example when we cited the ANSI article[2] in our editorial on updating the Standard Graphs in 2009.[1] Finally, and most important, our analysis finds the terminology in the original Alpins articles[4-6] to be superior by taking into account the strict mathematical and semantic context for the specific task of describing astigmatic vector changes in the ophthalmological domain. For clarity and reference, we have set out in Table 1 the original Alpins Method terms alongside the ANSI altered terms together with the reasoning behind the preference of adhering to the original terminology.

Since then, we were delighted to see that the *Journal of Cataract & Refractive Surgery*[15] has stated that they will also apply the standard as described by the 2014 *Journal of Refractive Surgery* editorial.[14] Furthermore, both the *Journal of Refractive Surgery* and the *Journal of Cataract & Refractive Surgery* have published an editorial using

Table 1
Terminology for Reporting Astigmatism

Alpins Method	ANSI	Reason
Target induced astigmatism vector (TIA)	Intended refractive correction	TIA is easily understood as the astigmatic correction that was attempted. On the other hand, the term "intended refractive correction" could also be interpreted as inclusive of sphere (eg as spherical equivalent).
Surgically induced astigmatism vector (SIA)	Surgically induced refractive correction (SIRC)	SIRC does not specifically apply to astigmatism (it can be misinterpreted as inclusive of sphere), whereas SIA can only be interpreted as the astigmatism achieved by the surgery. Also, SIA is a term that can be applied to either manifest refractive or corneal analysis, whereas SIRC would be inappropriate for corneal analysis alone.
Magnitude of error	Error of magnitude	This describes the arithmetic difference between the SIA and TIA (ie, the magnitude of the error). The term "error of magnitude" implies that the error is related to the magnitude of the treatment, which is not necessarily the case.
Angle of error	Error of angle	This describes the angle between the axis of the SIA and the axis of the TIA (ie, it is the angle of the error between these two vectors). It is not an error of an angle because by definition there are no angles in astigmatism (only axes); an angle does not specify a position in space, whereas an axis specifies the actual orientation.
Difference vector (DV)	Error vector	This is literally defined as the vectorial "difference" between the TIA and SIA vectors; this difference may not represent an "error" in the surgery or treatment because other factors could be in play causing such a "difference" to occur. In addition, the Alpins Method has precedence with no added benefit to changing the terminology.
Correction index	Correction ratio	This is defined as the SIA divided by the TIA. Although this could be described as either a ratio or an index, the Alpins Method has precedence with no added benefit to changing the terminology.
Index of success	Error ratio	This is defined as the DV divided by the TIA and provides the surgeon with a measure of the "success" in correcting the astigmatism rather than introducing the negative connotation of "error." In addition, the Alpins Method has precedence with no added benefit to changing the terminology.

Abbreviation: ANSI; American National Standards Institute.

the Alpins Method as a standard for reporting outcomes of intraocular lens surgery in 2017.[15,16] The clear position taken by the editorial boards of these journals will hopefully translate to a widespread phasing out of the ANSI report[2] terminology, and restoration of the original. To further help this process, I congratulate Noel on putting together a book that describes his entire methodology in one collection, and provides the reader with the tools to accurately analyze astigmatism.

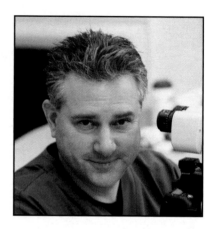

Dan Z. Reinstein, MD, MA(Cantab), FRCSC, DABO, FRCOphth, FEBO
London Vision Clinic, London, UK
Department of Ophthalmology
Columbia University Medical Center
New York City, New York
Centre Hospitalier National d'Ophtalmologie
Paris, France
Biomedical Science Research Institute
University of Ulster
Coleraine, Northern Ireland

References

1. Reinstein DZ, Waring GO, 3rd. Graphic Reporting of Outcomes of Refractive Surgery. *J Refract Surg.* 2009;25:975-978.

2. Eydelman MB, Drum B, Holladay J, Hilmantel G, Kezirian G, Durrie D, Stulting RD, Sanders D, Wong B. Standardized analyses of correction of astigmatism by laser systems that reshape the cornea. *J Refract Surg.* 2006;22:81-95.

3. Waring GO, 3rd. Review process for special articles [editor's comment]. *J Refract Surg.* 2006;22:529.

4. Alpins N. Astigmatism analysis by the Alpins method. *J Cataract Refract Surg.* 2001;27:31-49.

5. Alpins NA. Vector analysis of astigmatism changes by flattening, steepening, and torque. *J Cataract Refract Surg.* 1997;23:1503-1514.

6. Alpins NA. A new method of analyzing vectors for changes in astigmatism. *J Cataract Refract Surg.* 1993;19:524-533.

7. Alpins N. Terms used for the analysis of astigmatism. *J Refract Surg.* 2006;22:528; author reply 528-529.

8. Koch DD. Astigmatism analysis: the spectrum of approaches. *J Cataract Refract Surg.* 2006;32:1977-1978.

9. Kunert KS, Russmann C, Blum M, Sluyterman VLG. Vector analysis of myopic astigmatism corrected by femtosecond refractive lenticule extraction. *J Cataract Refract Surg.* 2013;39:759-769.

10. Schallhorn S, Brown M, Venter J, Teenan D, Hettinger K, Yamamoto H. Early clinical outcomes of wavefront-guided myopic LASIK treatments using a new-generation hartmann-shack aberrometer. *J Refract Surg.* 2014;30:14-21.

11. Alpins N. Vector analysis with the femtosecond laser. *J Cataract Refract Surg.* 2014;40:1246-1247.

12. Dupps WJ, Jr. Impact of citation practices: beyond journal impact factors. *J Cataract Refract Surg.* 2008;34:1419-1421.

13. Reinstein DZ, Archer TJ, Gobbe M. Combined corneal topography and corneal wavefront data in the treatment of corneal irregularity and refractive error in LASIK or PRK using the Carl Zeiss Meditec MEL80 and CRS Master. *J Refract Surg.* 2009;25:503-515.

14. Reinstein DZ, Archer TJ, Randleman JB. JRS Standard for Reporting Astigmatism Outcomes of Refractive Surgery. *J Refract Surg.* 2014;30:654-659.

15. Reinstein DZ, Archer TJ, Srinivasan S, et al. Standard for reporting refractive outcomes of intraocular lens-based refractive surgery. *J Refract Surg.* 2017;33(4):218-222.

16. Reinstein DZ, Archer TJ, Srinivasan S, et al. Standard for reporting refractive outcomes of intraocular lens-based refractive surgery. *J Cataract Refract Surg.* 2017;43(4); 435-439.

INTRODUCTION

My journey began in the mid 1980s, when I spent many clinical hours each week selectively removing sutures 4 weeks post-extracapsular cataract surgery to maximally reduce the magnitude of astigmatism and place it at a favorable orientation of with-the-rule. I realized then that there was a significant amount of mathematical and scientific evaluation required to quantify and improve astigmatic outcomes. I brought an excimer laser into my practice in 1991; soon after, I was struggling to understand how surgical astigmatic planning for incisional procedures, such as cataract incisions and astigmatic keratotomy, was based on the steepest corneal meridian and yet for refractive laser surgery involving the correction of astigmatism, the planning was based on manifest refraction alone without any regard for the astigmatism on the cornea, which in many cases was different in magnitude and/or orientation to the refractive cylinder.

The 1993 publication of a novel form of astigmatism analysis[1]—which came to be called the eponymous "Alpins Method"—sent me on a journey that cannot help but evoke the Grateful Dead: What a long, strange trip it's been.[2] I have circumnavigated the globe many times, spoke at many meetings, expanded my private practice, served on many editorial boards, reviewed and published many papers, and made great friends all over the world. I intend to continue the journey with all the appreciation and passion I can muster.

I have also described the Alpins Method to interested colleagues thousands of times. In many papers since 1993, the Alpins Method continues to be expanded and refined.

Here is the abstract from my 1993 paper:

This method of astigmatism analysis recognizes the need to define an astigmatism goal, thus allowing the surgeon to obtain precise, separate measures of the magnitude and the angle of surgical error. From this, the surgeon can evaluate what surgery may be required to achieve the initial preoperative goal. An index that measures correction that is adjusted for the level of preoperative astigmatism and a measure of success for comparative evaluation of results. The resulting data allow statistical comparison of multiple surgeries and techniques. This method also assists in resolving the case when spectacle and corneal astigmatism do not coincide.[1]

Understanding the Alpins Method is not an easy lift. Despite the fact that the basics of the method were described more than 20 years ago, I believe that far more ophthalmologists do not understand it versus the number who do. That is one of my incentives for writing this book—it will serve as a definitive, comprehensive, and accessible document on the Alpins Method and all the developments that have followed from it. It brings together into one volume all the writings I have published in the peer-reviewed literature, book chapters, and ophthalmic periodicals. This way, a deeper understanding of the techniques and how they interrelate with each other can be obtained. Most gratifyingly now, the Alpins Method has been adopted by our major journals as the standard means for study design and the reporting of results published in them.

I have never pretended that I invented the use of vector analysis apropos the cornea—this has been established well before my time; however, I do feel that I have taken analysis of vectors to new heights for both the corneal and refractive measures of astigmatism, and that my work helps put the eye-care community on the same page when it comes to planning and analyzing astigmatism associated with both refractive and cataract/intraocular lens surgery. I simply do not feel that a better way will be found for astigmatism analysis. I believe that the Alpins Method will continue to grow in importance, in concert with an increasing awareness of the method within the eye-care community.

References

1. Alpins NA. A new method of analyzing vectors for changes in astigmatism. *J Cataract Refract Surg.* 1993;19(4):524-533.
2. AllMusic Web site. http://www.allmusic.com/album/what-a-long-strange-trip-its-been-the-best-of-the-grateful-dead-mw0000198067. Accessed June 15, 2017.

Chapter 1

Astigmatism in the Population

DISTORTION BY DEFINITION

Astigmatism can be defined as a distortion of light entering the eye and coming to a focus at multiple points either in front of the retina, behind the retina, or both. Most commonly, astigmatism occurs due to an irregularly shaped cornea; less commonly, it is caused by the lens of the eye. Typically, an astigmatic cornea is asymmetrical—it is more curved along one meridian than the meridian 90° away. *Cylinder* is the refractive correction required to neutralize astigmatism. The subjective effect of astigmatism for the patient is a blurred and imperfect image.

If astigmatism did not exist, refractive surgery to correct myopia and hyperopia would be relatively straightforward. The practitioner would need only flatten (in the case of myopia) or steepen (in the case of hyperopia) corneal curvature to the proper degree to produce a focused image on the patient's retina. Planning, performance, and analysis of refractive surgery would be greatly simplified. Astigmatism, however, does exist, and it makes refractive, corneal and cataract/intraocular lens (IOL) surgery exponentially more complicated.

"INTERNAL" VERSUS "EXTERNAL" ASTIGMATISM

Astigmatism exists both within the eye—from the posterior cornea through the eye-brain interface—and on the anterior cornea. We have come to find that these two types of astigmatism are not necessarily aligned on the same meridian nor do they have the same magnitude.[1-3]

Other chapters in this book explore the discrepancy between internal and external astigmatism in detail. At this point, I will simply note that laser in situ keratomileusis (LASIK) and photoastigmatic refractive keratectomy (PARK) may be significantly less effective in correcting astigmatism that is mainly located in the internal optics[2]; and conversely, the efficacy of LASIK and PARK may be significantly higher in people whose

1

Alpins N. *Practical Astigmatism:*
Planning and Analysis (pp 1-6).
© 2018 SLACK Incorporated.

Figure 1-1. Polar diagram of irregular astigmatism, which would benefit from discrete laser treatment of each hemidivision.

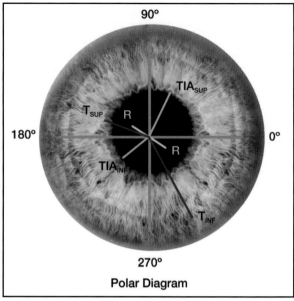

astigmatism is located mainly on the anterior corneal surface.[1-3] We have shown that about 7% of patients preoperatively have an internal astigmatism that could result in an increased post-LASIK astigmatism if ignored.[1]

Astigmatism became a major preoccupation of mine in the 1980s. I was vexed by the difficulty in recording and analyzing results in patients with astigmatism, as well as by the contradictory approaches between incisional procedures and, later in the 1990s at its inception, the laser—that is, incisional approaches were based on keratometry or topography of the anterior cornea and laser correction was based on refraction. My concentration on this problem led to the earliest description of my vector analysis approach in a 1993 publication.[4]

Other chapters of this book also describe my method for planning refractive surgery such that the astigmatic treatment is apportioned optimally between the refractive and topographic components, recognizing that a nonzero target exists and using its orientation as a guide to optimization.[1,5,6]

REGULAR VERSUS IRREGULAR ASTIGMATISM

In addition to its magnitude and meridian, astigmatism also may be classified based on its symmetry. Regular astigmatism is symmetric around the visual axis and classically shows a "bowtie" on corneal topography. The power of each meridian is successive as the meridians traverse 180°. Astigmatism that does not show symmetry or otherwise conforms to a geometric appearance is considered irregular astigmatism.

A Vector Planning approach can also be applied to the 2 corneal hemidivisions in patients with bowtie irregular astigmatism demonstrating asymmetry, a nonorthogonal relationship, or both (Figure 1-1). This allows a separate approach to each hemidivision, a capability that becomes more important as lasers are developed that can treat discrete portions of the cornea.[6]

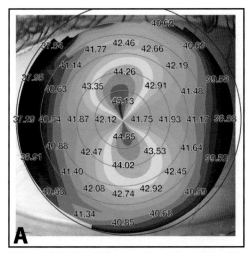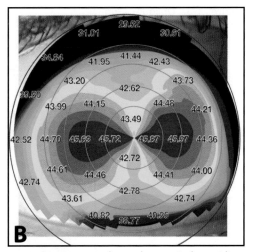

Figure 1-2. (A) With-the-rule astigmatism: The cornea is steepest along the vertical meridian. (B) Against-the-rule astigmatism: The cornea is steepest along the horizontal meridian.

WITH-THE-RULE, AGAINST-THE-RULE, AND OBLIQUE ASTIGMATISM

Astigmatism in its orientation may be classified as with-the-rule (WTR), against-the-rule (ATR), or oblique (Figures 1-2 and 1-3). WTR astigmatism is identified as the curvature of greatest power in the vertical meridian and the weakest power in the horizontal meridian. Therefore, WTR astigmatism has its flattest curve along the horizontal meridian; ATR astigmatism has its flattest curve along the vertical meridian.[7]

Oblique astigmatism (Figure 1-3) is a situation in which the two major meridia are at an intermediate axis other than horizontal or vertical. In oblique astigmatism, the greatest powers lie between 30° and 60°, and between 120° and 150°, or at 180° to these.[7]

Astigmatism may be corrected with eyeglasses, contact lenses, or refractive surgery[8] (glasses, however, do not adequately correct irregular astigmatism; rigid contact lenses are often prescribed for these patients).[7] In WTR astigmatism, a minus cylinder is placed in the horizontal axis (or a plus cylinder in the vertical axis). In ATR astigmatism, a plus cylinder is added in the horizontal axis (or a minus cylinder in the vertical axis).[8] This book does not further discuss the use of glasses or contact lenses in treating astigmatism, but instead concentrates on the laser and surgical approaches on the cornea and lens of interest to most cataract and refractive surgeons.

Children tend to have WTR astigmatism and elderly people tend to have ATR astigmatism.[8] WTR astigmatism is more common than ATR astigmatism.[7] In general, WTR astigmatism is visually more favorable than ATR astigmatism, and oblique astigmatism is the least favorable to perception.[6] The preference for WTR astigmatism in distance vision dates back to Javal's rule, published in 1890.[9]

Figure 1-3. Oblique astigmatism: Steepest curve is in oblique meridian along 120° to 150° or 30° to 60°.

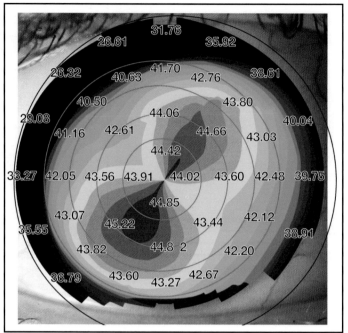

THE SIZE OF THE PROBLEM

Patients may experience astigmatism as blurred vision, often with streaks of light in dark conditions. Depending on the orientation, astigmatism also can cause tilting of the image. In general, patients will find 1 D or more of astigmatism to be significant, although some may find lesser amounts to be bothersome. One study suggests that as many as 20% of eyes with cataract have at least 1.5 D of corneal astigmatism.[10]

Most studies of refractive errors in large populations are based on manifest refraction.[11-14] Significant astigmatism, usually defined as cylinder of 1 D or greater, was seen in 10% to 50% of patients, differing with age and race/ethnicity.[12-16]

Probably the most important population-based study of refractive error was published in 2008, and included 12,010 patients culled from the large longitudinal National Health and Nutrition Examination Survey conducted between 1999 and 2004.[12] For people aged 20 or older, astigmatism of 1 D or greater was found in 36.2% (95% confidence interval of 34.9% to 37.5%). Figure 1-4 shows the total results by age and race/ethnicity.

These population-based studies convincingly demonstrate that the majority of people around the world have refractive errors. Additionally, astigmatism of a magnitude important to refractive and cataract surgeons is found in more than a third of prospective patients.[12-15,17]

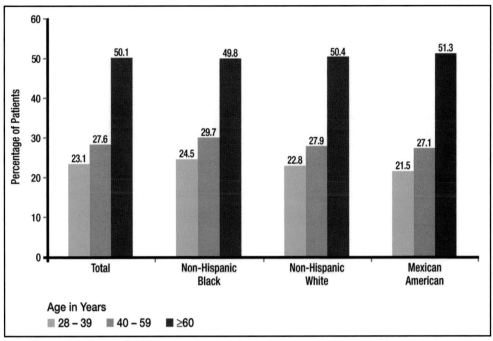

Figure 1-4. Prevalence of astigmatism (≥ 1 D cylinder) by age and race/ethnicity (%). (Adapted from Vitale S, Ellwein L, Cotch MF, Ferris FL III, Sperduto R. Prevalence of refractive error in the United States, 1999-2004. *Arch Ophthalmol*. 2008;126(8):1111-1119.)

REFERENCES

1. Alpins NA. New method of targeting vectors to treat astigmatism. *J Cataract Refract Surg*. 1997;23(1):65-75.

2. Qian YS, Huang J, Liu R, et al. Influence of internal optical astigmatism on the correction of myopic astigmatism by LASIK. *J Refract Surg*. 2011;27(12):863-868.

3. Kugler L, Cohen I, Haddad W, Wang MX. Efficacy of laser in situ keratomileusis in correcting anterior and non-anterior corneal astigmatism: comparative study. *J Cataract Refract Surg*. 2010;36(10):1745-1752.

4. Alpins NA. A new method of analyzing vectors for changes in astigmatism. *J Cataract Refract Surg*. 1993;19(4):524-533.

5. Alpins NA. Vector analysis of astigmatism changes by flattening, steepening, and torque. *J Cataract Refract Surg*. 1997;23(10):1503-1514.

6. Alpins N, Stamatelatos G. Chapter 24: The Cornea - Part X: Treatment and analysis of astigmatism during the laser era. In: Boyd BF, ed. *Modern Ophthalmology: The Highlights*. New Delhi, India: J.P. Medical Ltd; 2011:381-404.

7. Horner D, Thibos L. In: Wang M, ed. *Irregular Astigmatism: Diagnosis and Treatment*. Thorofare, NJ: SLACK Incorporated; 2008:9-22.

8. Carlton J. Basics and Beyond: Astigmatism Unraveling the mystery of this refractive error. Eyecare Business Web site. http://www.eyecarebusiness.com/issues/2013/september-2013/basics-and-beyond-astigmatism. Published September 1, 2013. Accessed June 25, 2017.

9. Javal E. *Memoires d'Ophthalmometrie*. Paris, France: G. Masson; 1890.

10. Hoffer KJ. Biometry of 7,500 cataractous eyes. *Am J Ophthalmol*. 1980;90(3):360-368.

11. Hashemi H, Khabazkhoob M, Peyman A, et al. The association between residual astigmatism and refractive errors in a population-based study. *J Refract Surg*. 2013;29(9):624-628.

12. Vitale S, Ellwein L, Cotch MF, Ferris FL III, Sperduto R. Prevalence of refractive error in the United States, 1999-2004. *Arch Ophthalmol.* 2008;126(8):1111-1119.

13. Wolfram C, Hohn R, Kottler U, et al. Prevalence of refractive errors in the European adult population: the Gutenberg Health Study (GHS). *Br J Ophthalmol.* 2014;98(7):857-861.

14. Pan CW, Klein BE, Cotch MF, et al. Racial variations in the prevalence of refractive errors in the United States: the multi-ethnic study of atherosclerosis. *Am J Ophthalmol.* 2013;155(6):1129-1138.

15. Yoo YC, Kim JM, Park KH, Kim CY, Kim TW. Refractive errors in a rural Korean adult population: the Namil Study. *Eye (Lond).* 2013;27(12):1368-1375.

16. Abrams D. Ophthalmic optics and refraction. In: Duke-Elder SS, ed. *System of Ophthalmology.* St Louis, MO: Mosby; 1970:671-674.

17. Buzard K, Shearing S, Relyea R. Incidence of astigmatism in a cataract practice. *J Refract Surg.* 1988;4:173-178.

Chapter 2

History of Vectorial Analysis of Astigmatism

SURGICAL CORRECTION OF ASTIGMATISM

In his doctoral thesis, published in 1898, Lans[1] evaluated patterns of keratotomy, keratectomy, and thermokeratoplasty, and defined some basic principles of astigmatic keratotomy. The thesis was titled "Experimental Studies of the Treatment of Astigmatism With Non-Perforating Corneal Incisions." Lans not only showed the flattening of the meridian perpendicular to a transverse incision but the steepening that occurred in the opposite meridian—the so-called coupling effect. He also discerned that longer and deeper incisions produced greater changes.

Thus, we know that the use of corneal incisions to correct astigmatism has a long history. Sato published an incisional method of astigmatic correction in 1939,[2] and Fyodorov in 1974.[3] Over the years, studies have been published on the use of corneal incisions to correct astigmatism related to keratoconus,[4] cataract/intraocular lens (IOL) surgery,[5,6] penetrating keratoplasty,[7] monocular diplopia,[8] and natural astigmatism.[9-12] In 1976, Barner described a number of surgical approaches to corneal astigmatism, concluding that the cresentic wedge resection was the most promising.[13] Sato's 1950 report[4] included the use of posterior corneal incisions for conical and irregular astigmatism; as is well known, posterior corneal incisions did not stand the test of time.

In the late 1970s into the 1980s, a number of other approaches were reported, including anterior keratotomies and "the dissection of the surgical ligament of the cornea."[14,15] In 1983, Sugar described relaxing keratotomies for postkeratoplasty high astigmatism.[7] A variation of radial keratotomy was even developed that corrected astigmatism.[10]

In the late 1980s arcuate keratotomies appeared, first reported in cadaver eyes[16] and then, clinically, after penetrating keratoplasty.[17] Lindstrom described his approach to

Alpins N. *Practical Astigmatism:*
Planning and Analysis (pp 7-15).
© 2018 SLACK Incorporated.

Figure 2-1. A typical pattern of arcuate keratotomies, made on the steepest corneal meridian, usually determined by keratometry.

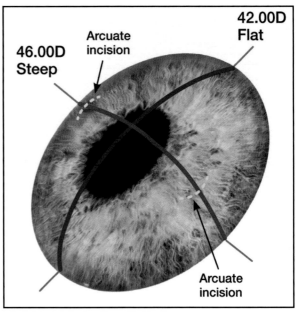

arcuate keratotomies in 1990.[18] Figure 2-1 shows a typical pattern of arcuate keratotomies, usually placed on the steepest meridian as determined by keratometry. Figure 2-2 shows transverse keratotomies placed on the steepest meridian in combination with a sutured incision for phacoemulsification and IOL implantation.[6] A combination of transverse and arcuate incisions was also described.[19]

WHAT IS A VECTOR?

A vector is a mathematical expression that combines values for magnitude and direction.[20] A vector cannot be measured, as one would measure the amount of astigmatism in diopters with an orientation using a manual keratometer. This is the fundamental difference in properties between astigmatisms and vectors. In the case of astigmatism analysis, vectors can only be calculated using values created or obtained by the various types of equipment that we use to measure astigmatism and cylinder—topographers, keratometers, wavefront aberrometers, autorefractors, etc.

For that reason, I have sometimes referred to vector analysis as reflecting the perfection of mathematics. If something goes wrong with a procedure—if we are surprised by the results, if we have undercorrected or overcorrected, or even if we hit the target and have a satisfied patient—it has nothing to do with the vector analysis involved. Either the equipment has over- or under-corrected, our procedure was flawed or was not performed as we had hoped, or the patient has demonstrated an idiosyncratic response to the surgery. If we hit the target and the patient is satisfied, again, that has nothing to do with the vector analysis (except in the case where we use vector analysis to initiate an alteration to a future procedure, with the intention of obtaining a different, improved result).

It is very seldom in life that we get a chance to describe something as perfect. Vector analysis has been used by many ophthalmologists, in many different ways, at many dif-

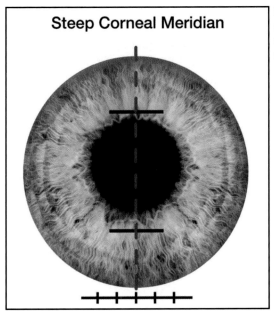

Steep Corneal Meridian

Figure 2-2. Transverse keratotomies placed on the steepest meridian (90°) in combination with sutured incision for phacoemulsification and intraocular lens implantation.

ferent times. Although I believe that some of these approaches may be more or less useful than others, all of them share one thing—the perfection of mathematics. One would be correct in concluding that I believe that the vector analysis methodology I have described over many years is more complete, more consistent and useful, and simply more evolved than any other vector approach described thus far when analyzing astigmatism.

ANALYZING THE RESULTS OF ASTIGMATIC INTERVENTION

As with many surgical procedures, no apparent "best" procedure for correcting astigmatism emerged in the early days of incisional astigmatism correction. A good surgeon with adequate experience could get good results, and as with many surgical procedures, the results would often get better as the surgeon gained experience—at least from the point of view of the patients reporting their subjective experience. Proper science, however, demands rigor and consistency. In the early days of surgical astigmatism correction, neither were available.

In 1993, I published my first paper on the use of vectors in astigmatism surgery, titled "A New Method of Analyzing Vectors for Changes in Astigmatism."[21] A number of my publications over the years have collectively come to be called the "Alpins Method."[20-25] Some aspects of the method have been patented,[26] and are programmed into a commercially available ophthalmic surgical analysis system, called ASSORT®[27] (Alpins Statistical System for Ophthalmic Refractive surgery Techniques), designed to help plan and analyze the results of refractive, corneal, and cataract surgical procedures.[24,28-35] The Alpins Method is detailed in later chapters. This chapter summarizes the Alpins Method in the context of other methods that have been used to analyze astigmatism and report astigmatic interventions in the literature.

THE VECTOR OF SURGICALLY INDUCED ASTIGMATISM

It is interesting to note that the classic formula for calculating surgically induced refractive change was published by Stokes in the mid-19th century.[36] Stokes' formula derives what is now called the surgically induced astigmatism vector (SIA) from the resultant lens by the addition in line of two planocylindrical lenses with different axes.

Prior to my 1993 paper,[21] methods had been described that could calculate the vector of change that was induced by a procedure, or the SIA. Investigators were able to determine the total induced astigmatism and the direction of the vector force acting in the eye and to calculate the mean total surgical astigmatism magnitude induced when a series of operations were compared. However, the axes of SIA usually varied considerably within the 0° to 180° range of arc, making it difficult to derive meaningful comparisons of astigmatic change for a series. An average directional change of vectors could not be calculated because vectors in opposing or partly opposing directions cancelled each other out in varying amounts. A summated vector mean provided some information about the net total SIA effect. My method solved those problems.

SUMMARY OF PRIOR RESEARCH

My 1993 report[21] as well as my other publications[20,25] cited much prior and/or relevant research. It is important to summarize them here to understand how I came to my understanding of vector analysis in astigmatism.

Hall et al,[37] and Merck et al,[38] both tabulated patient results individually, and neither were able to show a trend in induced astigmatism vectors as a group because the vectors had variable orientation. The respective approaches did not assess the success or desirability of the result, nor the extent to which the surgical goal was achieved.

Thornton and Sanders,[39] Neumann et al,[40] Maloney et al,[41] and Agapitos et al[42] attempted to correct the magnitude for the degree of axis change induced by tangential incisions by suggesting that this component varies as the cosine of the difference between the desired and the observed (achieved) axes. This corrected value of magnitude was substituted as the amount of surgically induced cylinder 90° to the axis of the incisions, considered the "proper" axis. Thornton and Sanders[39] incorporated Naylor's equations[43] into a computer program that essentially reproduced the Naylor table.

Naylor's report[43] included the first graphical representation of refractive cylinder on a double-angle plot where the angles of the astigmatism are doubled but the magnitude remains unchanged. In 1975, Jaffe and Clayman[44] described the use of rectangular and polar coordinates to determine, by vector analysis, the formula for calculating SIA and its axis using the known values of preoperative and postoperative corneal astigmatism. My method, for the first time, combined these approaches to address both corneal astigmatism and refractive cylinder.

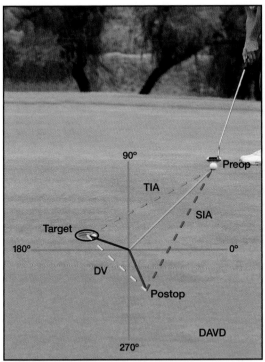

Figure 2-3. These are basic concepts of the Alpins Method, detailed in later chapters. Shown are the target induced astigmatism vector (TIA), the SIA, and the difference vector (DV), all of which have an analogue in a golf putt. The TIA represents the intended putt; the SIA represents the actual putt; and the DV represents a putt that would reach the golf cup on a second attempt. The values are calculated from (1) the patient's preoperative astigmatism; (2) the targeted astigmatism the surgeon plans to achieve; and (3) the actual achieved effect of the surgery. This vector analysis could be graphically represented using polar coordinates giving a more clinically relevant display, but is necessary to use a double-angle vector diagram, as shown here to calculate the vectors from astigmatism parameters.

Hall and coauthors[37] derived formulas analogous to those presented by Jaffe and Clayman[44] based on Martin and Welford's[45] derivation of Euler's theorem of curved surfaces: "The sum of the curvatures of any 2 perpendicular sections of a cylindrical or toric surface has a constant value." Euler's theorem is the link between Naeser's[46] and Jaffe and Clayman's[44] methods of vector analysis.

In 1992, Holladay and coauthors[47] calculated the surgically induced refractive change following surgery, but later described a flaw—the method presented for calculating the average axis or meridian of astigmatism was incorrect.[48]

A version of Figure 2-3 was presented in my original 1993 paper,[21] and is included here only to provide a sample of what is to come in this book. The figure succinctly captures concepts critical to understanding the Alpins Method approach and utility. Also included here (see Sidebars 2-1 and 2-2) is a glossary of indices and concepts that the reader may find helpful going forward.

Sidebar 2-1
Glossary of Indices Used in the Alpins Method

- **Correction index (CI)**—The ratio of the surgically induced astigmatism vector (SIA) to the target induced astigmatism vector (TIA)—what the surgery actually induced vs what the surgery was meant to induce. The CI is preferably 1; it is > 1 if an overcorrection occurs and < 1 if there is an undercorrection. The CI is calculated by dividing the SIA (actual effect) by the TIA (target effect).

- **Coefficient of adjustment (CA)**—The inverse of the CI, the CA quantifies the modification needed to the initial surgery plan to have achieved a CI of 1, the ideal correction. If the surgeon achieves an overcorrection—1.11, for example—the CA might be 0.9, indicating that the surgeon should have selected a correction 90% of what was actually selected. The CA can be used to refine nomograms for future procedures.

- **Magnitude of error (ME) and Angle of error (AE)**—The ME is the intended correction minus the actual correction in diopters. It is positive for an overcorrection and negative for an undercorrection of astigmatism. The AE is the angle described by the vectors of the intended correction vs the achieved correction (SIA minus TIA). By convention, the AE is positive if the achieved correction is on an axis counterclockwise to where it was intended, and negative if the achieved correction is clockwise to its intended axis.

    The ME and AE are calculated for, and directly comparable between, a series of multiple refractive surgery procedures and can determine the trend of a particular procedure. Mean and standard deviation values can be derived, allowing statistical analysis. These concepts separate the components of the operative error—magnitude and axis—and reveal the modifications that can be made to the original surgical plan in order to provide improved subsequent surgery.

- **Index of success (IOS)**—The IOS is calculated by dividing the DV (how far the target is missed) by the TIA (the original target effect). The IOS is a relative measure of success; that is, if golfer John attempts a long putt and golfer Bob attempts a shorter one, and each ends up the same distance from the cup, John's putt can be considered more successful because he had the longer initial putt and a lower IOS (zero being perfect). The IOS is a valuable measure of the relative effectiveness of various surgical procedures.

- **Flattening effect (FE)**—The amount of astigmatism reduction achieved at the intended treatment meridian; that is the effective portion of the SIA (FE = SIA cos2. AE).

- **Flattening index (FI)**—The FI is calculated by dividing the FE by the TIA and is preferably 1.0.

Sidebar 2-2
Concepts and Terms

- **Surgically induced astigmatism vector (SIA)**—The SIA is the amount and direction of corneal steepening that occurred in achieving the operative result from the preoperative astigmatic state. The SIA as used in the Alpins Method does not use the Law of Cosines, so that it is simpler to determine in which quadrant the coordinates lie.

  The SIA is the astigmatic change induced by any surgical procedure that alters the shape of the cornea. If the SIA coincides with the TIA vector (see below), the astigmatic goal of the surgery has been achieved. If the intention was for all the corneal astigmatism to be corrected, the SIA magnitude would equal that of the preoperative astigmatism, and their axes would be perpendicular to each other. If no change in the corneal astigmatism were intended (TIA of zero), the SIA would be equivalent to the magnitude of error.

- **Target induced astigmatism vector (TIA)**—The TIA is the amount and direction of the dioptric force required to achieve any desired astigmatic goal from any preoperative astigmatic state. When the astigmatic goal fails to coincide with the achieved result, the SIA and TIA do not coincide; they may vary in magnitude, axis, or both. When the SIA is greater than the TIA, an overcorrection has occurred; if less than the TIA, there has been an undercorrection. The greater the ratio of the TIA to the difference vector, the better the result achieved and the closer the index of success approaches zero. The TIA is the key to planning astigmatism surgery to achieve the astigmatic goal and resolve the dilemma occurring when corneal and spectacle astigmatism do not coincide. It provides a common parameter for analysis by any means of measuring astigmatism change and the calculated SIA.

- **Difference vector (DV)**—The DV represents the magnitude and axis of the difference in diopters between the desired operative result and the result achieved. The axis is half that subtended when calculated on the 360° double angle vector diagram; by placing its magnitude on a 180° chart, it would describe the dioptric correction (the amount of steepening and its axis) required for a secondary operation to achieve the targeted goal for that eye. However, the DV should not be used as a parameter for retreatment, as it is more of a score card to gauge the absolute success of surgery not related to the amount of the treatment; the treatment parameters for an enhancement would need to be based on remeasured refractive and corneal parameters.

  The DV is specific to the one eye in which it is calculated. The DV can provide a valuable basis for statistical analysis between multiple operations. The magnitude of the DV gives a measure of the total dioptric distance between the desired and the achieved results. It is independent of the TIA and therefore, does not relate the success of surgery to the initial amount of desired correction. When the difference vector is zero, the index of success is also zero, indicating the astigmatic goal has been achieved. The mean magnitude of the DV and the summated vector mean of the DV provide valuable information on any trends existing in a series of surgeries.

REFERENCES

1. Lans LJ. Experimentelle Untersuchungen über Entstehung von Astigmatismus durch nich-perfori-rende Corneawunden. *Graefes Arch Ophthalmol.* 1898;45:117.

2. Sato T. Treatment of conical cornea (incision of Descemet's membrane). *Acta Societatis Ophthalmologicae Japonicae.* 1939;43:544-555.

3. Political parties and their leaders: Russian presidential candidates 1996: Fyodorov Svyatoslav Nikolayevich. Panorama Web site. http://www.panorama.ru/works/oe/fyodoroe.html. Accessed April 1, 2014.

4. Sato T. Posterior incision of cornea; surgical treatment for conical cornea and astigmatism. *Am J Ophthalmol.* 1950;33(6):943-948.

5. Jensen RP, Jensen AC. Surgical correction of astigmatism by microwedge resection of the limbus. *Ophthalmology.* 1978;85(12):1288-1298.

6. Osher RH. Paired transverse relaxing keratotomy: a combined technique for reducing astigmatism. *J Cataract Refract Surg.* 1989;15(1):32-37.

7. Sugar J, Kirk AK. Relaxing keratotomy for post-keratoplasty high astigmatism. *Ophthalmic Surg.* 1983;14(2):156-158.

8. Records RE. Monocular diplopia. *Surv Ophthalmol.* 1980;24(5):303-306.

9. Fyodorov SN, Puchkov SG. Chemical and mechanical influence of intraocular lenses on rabbit eye tissue. *Ann Ophthalmol.* 1981;13(11):1259-1264.

10. Grady FJ. Radial keratotomy for astigmatism. *Ann Ophthalmol.* 1984;16(10):942-944.

11. Pavilack MA, Halpem BL. Effectiveness of incisional keratotomy for moderate to high astigmatism. *Investigative Ophthalmology and Visual Science.* 1996;37(3):S661.

12. Price FW, Grene RB, Marks RG, Gonzales JS. Astigmatism reduction clinical trial: a multicenter prospective evaluation of the predictability of arcuate keratotomy. Evaluation of surgical nomogram predictability. ARC-T Study Group. *Arch Ophthalmol.* 1995;113(3):277-282.

13. Barner SS. Surgical treatment of corneal astigmatism. *Ophthalmic Surg.* 1976;7(1):43-48.

14. Fyodorov SN, Durnev VV. [Surgical correction of complex myopic astigmatism by means of anterior keratotomy]. *Oftalmol Zh.* 1979;34(4):210-213.

15. Fyodorov SN, Durnev VV. Surgical correction of complicated myopic astigmatism by means of dis-section of circular ligament of cornea. *Ann Ophthalmol.* 1981;13(1):115-118.

16. Duffey RJ, Jain VN, Tchah H, Hofmann RF, Lindstrom RL. Paired arcuate keratotomy. A surgical approach to mixed and myopic astigmatism. *Arch Ophthalmol.* 1988;106(8):1130-1135.

17. Cohen KL, Tripoli NK, Noecker RJ. Prospective analysis of photokeratoscopy for arcuate keratotomy to reduce postkeratoplasty astigmatism. *Refract Corneal Surg.* 1989;5(6):388-393.

18. Lindstrom RL. The surgical correction of astigmatism: a clinician's perspective. *Refract Corneal Surg.* 1990;6(6):441-454.

19. Thornton SP. Theory behind corneal relaxing incisions/Thornton nomogram. In: Gills JP, Martin RG, Sanders DR, ed. *Sutureless Cataract Surgery.* Thorofare, NJ: SLACK Incorporated; 1992:123-144.

20. Alpins NA, Goggin M. Practical astigmatism analysis for refractive outcomes in cataract and refrac-tive surgery. *Surv Ophthalmol.* 2004;49(1):109-122.

21. Alpins NA. A new method of analyzing vectors for changes in astigmatism. *J Cataract Refract Surg.* 1993;19(4):524-533.

22. Alpins NA. New method of targeting vectors to treat astigmatism. *J Cataract Refract Surg.* 1997;23(1):65-75.

23. Alpins NA. Vector analysis of astigmatism changes by flattening, steepening, and torque. *J Cataract Refract Surg.* 1997;23(10):1503-1514.

24. Alpins N, Stamatelatos G. Clinical outcomes of laser in situ keratomileusis using combined topography and refractive wavefront treatments for myopic astigmatism. *J Cataract Refract Surg.* 2008;34(8):1250-1259.

25. Alpins N, Stamatelatos G. Chapter 24: The Cornea - Part X: Treatment and analysis of astigmatism during the laser era. In: Boyd BF, ed. *Modern Ophthalmology: The Highlights.* New Delhi, India: J.P. Medical Ltd; 2011:381-404.

26. Noel Alpins Patent Search Results. Google Web site. https://www.google.com/search?q=Noel+Alpins&btnG=Search+Patents&tbm=pts&tbo=1&hl=en. Accessed April 22, 2014.

27. ASSORT Web site. http://www.assort.com. Accessed April 22, 2014.

28. Alpins NA, Tabin GC, Adams LM, Aldred GF, Kent DG, Taylor HR. Refractive versus corneal changes after photorefractive keratectomy for astigmatism. *J Refract Surg.* 1998;14(4):386-396.

29. Fraenkel GE, Webber SK, Sutton GL, Lawless MA, Rogers CM. Toric laser in situ keratomileusis for myopic astigmatism using an ablatable mask. *J Refract Surg.* 1999;15(2):111-117.

30. Alpins N, Stamatelatos G. Customized photoastigmatic refractive keratectomy using combined topographic and refractive data for myopia and astigmatism in eyes with forme fruste and mild keratoconus. *J Cataract Refract Surg.* 2007;33(4):591-602.

31. Pinero DP, Alio JL, Teus MA, Barraquer RI, Michael R, Jimenez R. Modification and refinement of astigmatism in keratoconic eyes with intrastromal corneal ring segments. *J Cataract Refract Surg.* 2010;36(9):1562-1572.

32. Alio JL, Agdeppa MC, Pongo VC, El KB. Microincision cataract surgery with toric intraocular lens implantation for correcting moderate and high astigmatism: pilot study. *J Cataract Refract Surg.* 2010;36(1):44-52.

33. Galway G, Drury B, Cronin BG, Bourke RD. A comparison of induced astigmatism in 20- vs 25-gauge vitrectomy procedures. *Eye (Lond).* 2010;24(2):315-317.

34. Alio JL, Pinero DP, Tomas J, Plaza AB. Vector analysis of astigmatic changes after cataract surgery with implantation of a new toric multifocal intraocular lens. *J Cataract Refract Surg.* 2011;37(7):1217-1229.

35. Alio JL, Pinero DP, Tomas J, Aleson A. Vector analysis of astigmatic changes after cataract surgery with toric intraocular lens implantation. *J Cataract Refract Surg.* 2011;37(6):1038-1049.

36. Stokes GG. On a mode of measuring the astigmatism of a defective eye. *Transactions of the 19th meeting of the British Association for the Advancement of Science 1849.* London, England: British Association for the Advancement of Science; 1850.

37. Hall GW, Campion M, Sorenson CM, Monthofer S. Reduction of corneal astigmatism at cataract surgery. *J Cataract Refract Surg.* 1991;17(4):407-414.

38. Merck MP, Williams PA, Lindstrom RL. Trapezoidal keratotomy. A vector analysis. *Ophthalmology.* 1986;93(6):719-726.

39. Thornton SP, Sanders DR. Graded nonintersecting transverse incisions for correction of idiopathic astigmatism. *J Cataract Refract Surg.* 1987;13(1):27-31.

40. Neumann AC, McCarty GR, Sanders DR, Raanan MG. Refractive evaluation of astigmatic keratotomy procedures. *J Cataract Refract Surg.* 1989;15(1):25-31.

41. Maloney WF, Sanders DR, Pearcy DE. Astigmatic keratotomy to correct preexisting astigmatism in cataract patients. *J Cataract Refract Surg.* 1990;16(3):297-304.

42. Agapitos PJ, Lindstrom RL, Williams PA, Sanders DR. Analysis of astigmatic keratotomy. *J Cataract Refract Surg.* 1989;15(1):13-18.

43. Naylor EJ. Astigmatic difference in refractive errors. *Br J Ophthalmol.* 1968;52(5):422-425.

44. Jaffe NS, Clayman HM. The pathophysiology of corneal astigmatism after cataract extraction. *Transactions of the American Academy of Ophthalmology and Otolaryngology.* Rochester, MN: 1975:OP-615-OP-630.

45. Martin LC, Welford WT. Technical Optics. 2nd ed. London, England: Pitman Publishing; 1966.

46. Naeser K. Conversion of keratometer readings to polar values. *J Cataract Refract Surg.* 1990;16(6):741-745.

47. Holladay JT, Cravy TV, Koch DD. Calculating the surgically induced refractive change following ocular surgery. *J Cataract Refract Surg.* 1992;18(5):429-443.

48. Holladay JT, Dudeja DR, Koch DD. Evaluating and reporting astigmatism for individual and aggregate data. *J Cataract Refract Surg.* 1998;24(1):57-65.

Chapter 3

A Dilemma
The Conflict Between Incisional and Laser Ablative Approaches

ASTIGMATIC KERATOTOMY IN THE MODERN ERA

Building on the work of pioneers such as Sato[1] and Fyodorov,[2] modern astigmatic keratotomy developed into what it is today via two historical paths: corneal transplantation and radial keratotomy.[3] The era of refractive surgery during which radial keratotomy was widely practiced—and, indeed, considered state of the art—actually provided the impetus for the creation and improvement of tools such as diamond blades and knives, markers, and pachymeters.

By the 1990s, there were three main schools of astigmatic keratotomy,[3] which form the basis of modern incisional astigmatic approaches.

The Nordan School

Nordan's surgical approach[4] (Figure 3-1) is the simplest of the three, utilizing transverse incisions, a single optical zone (7 mm), a goal for incision depth of 80% to 90%, a coupling ratio of 2:1, and no modifications for the age of the patient.

The Lindstrom School

Lindstrom's approach to incisional astigmatism treatment (Figure 3-2) formed the basis of the ARC-T (astigmatism reduction clinical trial) study.[5] The approach assumed a 1.5 coupling ratio[6] and a significant age factor. Lindstrom's use of arcuate incisions was based on work by Merlin[7]; the technique corrected between 1 D and 7.5 D of astigmatism, depending on the patient's age.

The ARC-T study found that the original Lindstrom surgical nomogram tended to under-predict results, especially in older patients and in patients who received two incisions.[5]

Alpins N. *Practical Astigmatism:*
Planning and Analysis (pp 17-25).
© 2018 SLACK Incorporated.

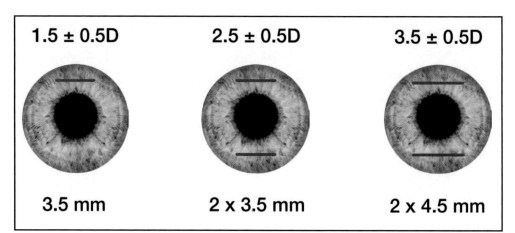

Figure 3-1. The Nordan nomogram utilized a single optical zone of 7 mm. (Adapted from Grene RB, Lindstrom RL. Astigmatic keratotomy in the refractive patient: the ARC-T study. In: Gills JP, Martin RG, Thornton SP, Sanders DR, eds. *Surgical Treatment of Astigmatism*. Thorofare, NJ: SLACK Incorporated; 1994:11-26.)

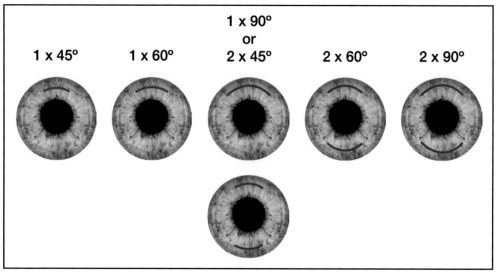

Figure 3-2. Options used in the ARC-T study. The ARC-T study found that the most significant predictors of the magnitude of achieved astigmatic correction were the number of incisions, incision length, age, and gender (in order of importance). (Adapted from Grene RB, Lindstrom RL. Astigmatic keratotomy in the refractive patient: the ARC-T study. In: Gills JP, Martin RG, Thornton SP, Sanders DR, eds. *Surgical Treatment of Astigmatism*. Thorofare, NJ: SLACK Incorporated; 1994:11-26.)

The ARC-T study design did not employ the Alpins Method in data analysis.[5] The Holladay-Cravy-Koch vector analysis method was used instead. However, in a 1994 book, Grene and Lindstrom compared the four vector analysis approaches then available, which included the Alpins Method. The authors noted that the Alpins Method introduced helpful "evaluatory aids," such as target induced astigmatism vector (TIA) and difference vector (DV), and was the only vector analysis approach to calculate the correct angular component.[3]

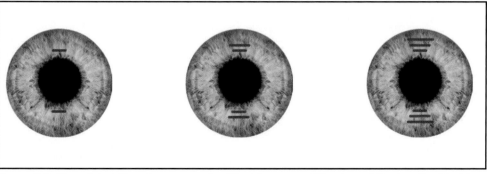

Figure 3-3. The original Thornton approach utilized transverse (T) cuts, and the length of incisions varied depending on the desired correction. The optical zone (OZ) for 1 pair (left) was 7 mm; the OZs for 2 pairs (center) were 6 mm and 8 mm; and the OZs for 3 pairs (right) were 6 mm, 7 mm, and 8 mm. The T-cut nomogram also modified these characteristics depending on the patient's age and intraocular pressure. (Adapted from Grene RB, Lindstrom RL. Astigmatic keratotomy in the refractive patient: the ARC-T study. In: Gills JP, Martin RG, Thornton SP, Sanders DR, eds. *Surgical Treatment of Astigmatism*. Thorofare, NJ: SLACK Incorporated; 1994:11-26.)

The Thornton School

Thornton's approach[8,9] originally employed transverse (T) incisions, but he later articulated a detailed nomogram based on arcuate incisions.[8] The T-cut approach is shown in Figure 3-3.

Astigmatic keratotomy consisting of arcuate incisions—which have been found to flatten the steeper meridian about the same amount as they steepen the flatter meridian, hence, a coupling ratio of 1.0—at a 9-mm optical zone is today a widely used approach. Arcuate incisions > 90° are usually avoided because they risk late wound dehiscence.[10]

The Nordan, Lindstrom, and Thornton schools of astigmatic keratotomy, and the variations that have evolved from them, share a notable feature: for patients with regular astigmatism, the incisions are placed on the steep corneal meridian.

ALONG CAME THE LASER

When performed today, astigmatic keratotomy is most commonly done:
- At the time or after cataract surgery, where the approach is often referred to as limbal relaxing incisions.
- To correct astigmatism after corneal transplantation.

Its use is becoming less common due to good results with astigmatic laser correction and the wide availability of ablative lasers. The increasing use of toric intraocular lens implants also may contribute to the decreasing use of incisional astigmatic techniques.[11]

An excimer laser reduces simple myopia by exposing the central cornea to more laser energy than the peripheral cornea.[12-14] For a static laser light, this is done by opening and closing a circular aperture between the laser source and the cornea. In the case of a scanning laser, laser pulses are simply directed in a pattern that provides overall greater exposure at the central cornea. Both mechanisms result in a relatively deeper ablation of the central stromal tissue vs the peripheral stromal tissue, creating an overall flattening of

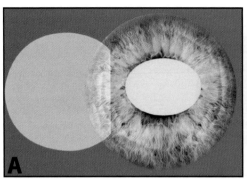 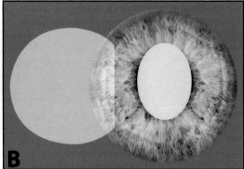

Figure 3-4. (A) LASIK ablation patterns are shown for myopic with-the-rule astigmatism and (B) myopic against-the-rule astigmatism. Both ablations induce a flattening along the steep meridian or short axis.

the cornea.[14,15] Hyperopic corrections are achieved by mechanisms whereby tissue in the peripheral cornea receives more laser energy than tissue in the central cornea.

Myopic astigmatic corrections are achieved by applying the laser energy in an elliptical pattern along the central part of the flat meridian, thereby relatively flattening the steep meridian.[10] Figure 3-4 shows the ablation patterns for myopic with-the-rule and against-the-rule astigmatism.

Alternatively, hyperopic astigmatic corrections are achieved by applying the laser energy preferentially in the periphery, steepening the flat meridian (Figure 3-5).

With few exceptions, ophthalmic surgeons and laser manufacturers recommend that laser ablative correction should be sculpted onto the cornea based on the patient's manifest refraction.[16-18]

INTEGRATING THE DICHOTOMY

When I first began to practice ophthalmology, much of my motivation came from the idea of providing people with better eyesight. This goal prompted me to develop the Alpins Method of astigmatism analysis and the many related papers and studies with which I have been involved over my career (Sidebar 3-1). Additonally, my enthusiasm for improving the vision of my patients has only grown over time.

As described in Chapter 2, the science of surgical astigmatism treatment and analysis in the late 1980s through the early 1990s was imperfect and limited. I believe that many thoughtful ophthalmic surgeons at the time recognized the contradiction that existed between incisional and laser approaches—that is, the use of incisions straddling the steep corneal meridian as identified by corneal shape (keratometry or topography) vs the use of astigmatic laser treatment based on refractive cylinder. The obvious dilemma: How can there be two different surgical paradigms to achieve the same goal of astigmatism reduction and improved unaided vision? Some leading ophthalmic surgeons even found themselves in both camps at the same time!

A manifest refraction identifies the myopic or hyperopic correction, as well as the magnitude and axis of total astigmatic correction needed for clear vision. However, as with the patient shown in Figure 3-6, most people with astigmatism demonstrate differ-

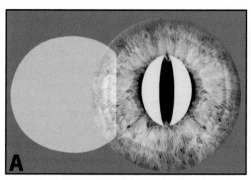
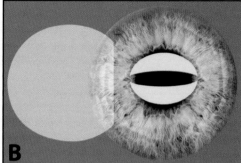

Figure 3-5. (A) LASIK for hyperopic with-the-rule astigmatism and (B) hyperopic against-the-rule astigmatism.

Sidebar 3-1
The People Who Made a Difference

Throughout this book, I will be recalling the personalities and events that helped guide me through a long, exciting, and satisfying career. Not all of these people and events, whether intentionally or not, exerted a positive influence. Fortunately, adversity carries just as many lessons as success does—perhaps more.

Of course, my wife, Sylvia, was a huge (positive) influence early in my life and career. There were countless hours spent on astigmatism planning and analysis to finally decide on the Alpins Method, and Sylvia was always by my side.

Even before Sylvia, though, there was Hugh Taylor—a well-known Australian ophthalmologist. Hugh and I were in grade 2 together, and proceeded to live weirdly parallel lives. Academically, we were equivalent to the point that we could not be singled out or broken up. I recall a contest of some sort in which we tied for fourth place in second grade. A bit frustrated, the teacher was forced to award us both the same prize—a book called *Fairy Tales of Long Ago*, which I still have. I would be willing to bet a good amount that Hugh has held on to his copy too.

Many, many people helped me with the concepts, the mathematical constructs, the faculty and speaking invitations, the studies and journal articles, and the ever-expanding applications of my work on a vector analysis approach to astigmatism. It will be my pleasure to name those who, over the years, have honored me with their ideas, encouragement, selflessness, and friendship.

As I recount in this chapter, my early dilemma reconciling corneal vs refractive astigmatism as a basis for incisional and ablative correction, respectively, I think of skiing in 1991, at a meeting in Aspen, Colorado. I met Steve Siepser there, and though I was not part of the faculty, after talking with Steve, he offered to help get me invited to speak at the next Aspen meeting. Later in 1991, he came to Melbourne and stayed with us for a couple of days. Soon after, I received my first invitation to speak—at the Aspen meeting scheduled for early 1992. In preparation for that presentation, I began to analyze my data, sought out a computer programmer to help me, and analyzed vectors of the various phacoemulsification incisions I had been using for several years. The 1992 Aspen meeting convened by David Dulaney was the impetus for me to begin appreciating the complexity of astigmatism and the many holes I had to fill, and it put me on the road to developing the Alpins Method.

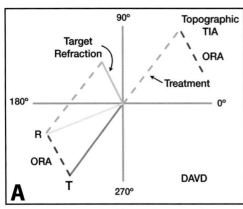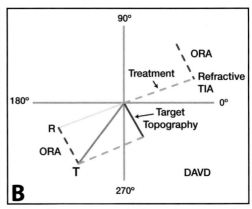

Figure 3-6. These double-angle vector diagrams (DAVDs) show a patient who has a discrepancy between refractive (R) and corneal topographic (T) astigmatism. The vector connecting R and T and directed towards R is the ORA—the minimal amount of astigmatism that can remain in the optical system of this eye. If the patient's targeted treatment is based 100% on T (A), the target refraction is the amount of refractive astigmatism remaining after treatment to eliminate topographic astigmatism—that is, the cornea would be spherical but the patient would have a remaining refractive astigmatism equal to the target refraction (and ORA) shown. The treatment is shown as a vector of equivalent magnitude to T, but directed 180° away from T on the DAVD. In the DAVD on the right (B), the correction is targeted 100% on refractive cylinder. The target topography is the corneal topographic astigmatism remaining after treatment to eliminate the refractive astigmatism. The treatment vector has an equivalent magnitude to R, but is directed 180° away from R on the DAVD (actual steepening treatment on the cornea would be 90° away).

ences in magnitude and axis between corneal topographic astigmatism (T) and positive refractive cylinder (R).[16] As will be described in greater detail in Chapter 9, the inherent difference between T and R result in our inability as surgeons to fully eliminate astigmatism from the refractive system of the eye.[16,17,19] In a perfect world, refractive cylinder and corneal astigmatism would be identical in magnitude and orientation and the dilemma would be nonexistent.

Intro to Ocular Residual Astigmatism

The vectorial difference between the corneal astigmatism and the refractive cylinder (at the corneal plane) is known as ocular residual astigmatism (ORA), and is expressed in diopters. ORA is the astigmatism in the eye not attributable to the anterior corneal surface.[20,21] (Note—ORA is distinct from what is sometimes called residual astigmatism or surgical residual astigmatism, which is the astigmatism remaining after surgery.) ORA is also called intraocular, internal, lenticular, or noncorneal astigmatism. ORA is the minimal amount of astigmatism that can remain in the overall optical system of the eye[18,22-25] regardless of how perfect the surgical procedure was performed.

For the patient shown in Figure 3-6, an intermediate TIA vector can be chosen between the boundaries of the topographic TIA and the refractive TIA (Figure 3-7). The relative proximity of the intersection to either the topographic or refractive end points (heavy dashed line) is determined by the emphasis of treatment required (total will equal 100%). Any TIA that achieves the minimum target astigmatism for the prevailing topographic and refractive parameters will terminate on the ORA line. The Alpins Method

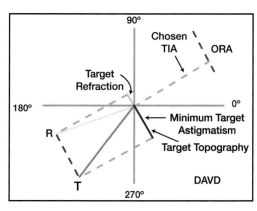

Figure 3-7. A double-angle vector diagram of the same patient in Figure 3-6. In this case, the treatment emphasis is divided between refractive (R) and topographic (T) astigmatism. Any TIA that achieves the minimum target astigmatism for the prevailing topographic and refractive parameters will terminate on the ORA line being the maximal treatment for the minimum remaining astigmatism.

offers a rationale for choosing a preferred treatment emphasis, which favors a postoperative corneal astigmatism that is with-the-rule.

Laser in situ keratomileusis (LASIK) is significantly less effective in correcting astigmatism when astigmatism is predominantly located in the internal optics[26]—that is, a patient with high ORA—and conversely, the efficacy of LASIK is significantly higher in people whose astigmatism is located mainly on the anterior corneal surface[24-28]—that is, patients with low ORA.

About 7% of patients preoperatively have an ORA that could result in increased post-LASIK corneal astigmatism compared to what prevailed prior to surgery.[16] It is likely that unrecognized high preoperative ORA is responsible for many unhappy LASIK patients.[22] People with high preoperative ORA can be better managed if their expectations are lowered as to their postoperative results and/or they are treated using a Vector Planning approach, which optimizes postoperative results using a combination of both refractive and corneal parameters.

Wavefront and Vector Analysis: Good Partners

In the early 2000s, wavefront technology was seen as a possible "holy grail" that could provide "super vision" for refractive surgery patients.[27-30] I queried its benefits in *Ocular Surgery News* articles in 2000[29,30] and in 2001.[28] In an invited editorial in 2002,[31] I raised questions on the capability of wavefront technology to solve the dilemma of corneal vs refractive astigmatism correction, creating excess regular and irregular astigmatism with the wavefront-guided ablation. In those publications and others, I pointed out the importance of combining the Vector Planning approach, seldom used at the time, with the then-standard use of corneal topography or optical/refractive measurements.[29-31]

This prediction was confirmed in a small, prospective, masked study that we published in 2008 (21 eyes in 14 patients receiving LASIK).[32] We found a greater reduction in corneal astigmatism and better visual outcomes under mesopic conditions using wavefront technology combined with a Vector Planning approach than using wavefront technology alone, and also found equivalent higher-order aberrations.[32,33] Noting this study, other investigators have acknowledged that a combined approach will be "the treatment approach of the future."[26,34]

REFERENCES

1. Sato T. Posterior incision of cornea; surgical treatment for conical cornea and astigmatism. *Am J Ophthalmol.* 1950;33(6):943-948.

2. Fyodorov SN, Durnev VV. Surgical correction of complicated myopic astigmatism by means of dissection of circular ligament of cornea. *Ann Ophthalmol.* 1981;13(1):115-118.

3. Grene RB, Lindstrom RL. Astigmatic keratotomy in the refractive patient: the ARC-T study. In: Gills JP, Martin RG, Thornton SP, Sanders DR, eds. *Surgical Treatment of Astigmatism.* Thorofare, NJ: SLACK Incorporated; 1994:11-26.

4. Nordan LT. Quantifiable astigmatism correction: concepts and suggestions, 1986. *J Cataract Refract Surg.* 1986;12(5):507-518.

5. Price FW, Grene RB, Marks RG, Gonzales JS. Astigmatism reduction clinical trial: a multicenter prospective evaluation of the predictability of arcuate keratotomy. Evaluation of surgical nomogram predictability. ARC-T Study Group. *Arch Ophthalmol.* 1995;113(3):277-282.

6. Duffey RJ, Jain VN, Tchah H, Hofmann RF, Lindstrom RL. Paired arcuate keratotomy. A surgical approach to mixed and myopic astigmatism. *Arch Ophthalmol.* 1988;106(8):1130-1135.

7. Merlin U. Curved keratotomy procedure for congenital astigmatism. *J Refract Surg.* 1987;3:92-97.

8. Grabow HB. Cataract with corneal astigmatism. In: Roy FH, Arzabe CW, eds. *Master Techniques in Cataract and Refractive Surgery.* Thorofare, NJ: SLACK Incorporated; 2004:47-61.

9. Thornton SP, Sanders DR. Graded nonintersecting transverse incisions for correction of idiopathic astigmatism. *J Cataract Refract Surg.* 1987;13(1):27-31.

10. Hardten DR, Roy R. LASIK astigmatism treatment and management. Medscape Web site. http://emedicine.medscape.com/article/1220489-treatment#a1128. Accessed August 5, 2014.

11. Lee WB. Astigmatic keratotomy recovery. American Academy of Ophthalmology EyeSmart Web site. http://www.geteyesmart.org/eyesmart/ask/questions/astigmatic-keratotomy.cfm. Accessed August 4, 2014.

12. Linebarger EJ, Hardten DR, Lindstrom RL. Sands of the Sahara. In: Burratto L, Brint S, eds. *LASIK: Surgical Techniques and Complications.* Thorofare, NJ: SLACK Incorporated; 2014:591-596.

13. Munnerlyn CR, Koons SJ, Marshall J. Photorefractive keratectomy: a technique for laser refractive surgery. *J Cataract Refract Surg.* 1988;14(1):46-52.

14. Trokel SL, Srinivasan R, Braren B. Excimer laser surgery of the cornea. *Am J Ophthalmol.* 1983;96(6):710-715.

15. Shah S, Smith RJ, Pieger S, Chatterjee A. Effect of an elliptical optical zone on outcome of photoastigmatic refractive keratectomy. *J Refract Surg.* 1999;15(2 Suppl):S188-S191.

16. Alpins NA. New method of targeting vectors to treat astigmatism. *J Cataract Refract Surg.* 1997;23(1):65-75.

17. Alpins NA. Corneal versus refractive astigmatism: integrated analysis. *Ocular Surgery News.* June 15, 1999:44.

18. Alpins NA, Terry CM. Astigmatism: LASIK, LASEK, and PRK. In: Roy FH, Arzabe CW, eds. *Master Techniques in Cataract and Refractive Surgery.* Thorofare, NJ: SLACK Incorporated; 2004:151-60.

19. Alpins NA. A new method of analyzing vectors for changes in astigmatism. *J Cataract Refract Surg.* 1993;19(4):524-533.

20. Alpins N, Stamatelatos G. Customized photoastigmatic refractive keratectomy using combined topographic and refractive data for myopia and astigmatism in eyes with forme fruste and mild keratoconus. *J Cataract Refract Surg.* 2007;33(4):591-602.

21. Lyle WM. Changes in corneal astigmatism with age. *Am J Optom Arch Am Acad Optom.* 1971;48(6):467-478.

22. Alio JL, Alpins N. Excimer laser correction of astigmatism: consistent terminology for better outcomes. *J Refract Surg.* 2014;30(5):294-295.

23. Alpins NA. Vector analysis of astigmatism changes by flattening, steepening, and torque. *J Cataract Refract Surg.* 1997;23(10):1503-1514.

24. Frings A, Katz T, Steinberg J, Druchkiv V, Richard G, Linke SJ. Ocular residual astigmatism: effects of demographic and ocular parameters in myopic laser in situ keratomileusis. *J Cataract Refract Surg.* 2014;40(2):232-238.

25. Martinez-Abad A, Pinero DP, Ruiz-Fortes P, Artola A. Evaluation of the diagnostic ability of vector parameters characterizing the corneal astigmatism and regularity in clinical and subclinical keratoconus. *Cont Lens Anterior Eye.* 2017;40(2):88-96.

26. Qian YS, Huang J, Liu R, et al. Influence of internal optical astigmatism on the correction of myopic astigmatism by LASIK. *J Refract Surg.* 2011;27(12):863-868.

27. Archer TJ, Reinstein DZ, Pinero DP, Gobbe M, Carp GI. Comparison of the predictability of refractive cylinder correction by laser in situ keratomileusis in eyes with low or high ocular residual astigmatism. *J Cataract Refract Surg.* 2015;41(7):1383-1392.

28. Alpins NA. At Issue: Custom corneal ablations. Optimistic but marginal improvement. Ocular Surgery News Web site. http://www.healio.com/ophthalmology/refractive-surgery/news/print/ocular-surgery-news/%7B4ed75290-205f-45fd-9bcf-58c6d4eabf30%7D/at-issue-custom-corneal-ablations. Accessed September 15, 2014.

29. Walsh MJ. Is the future of refractive surgery based on corneal topography or wavefront? Ocular Surgery News Web site. http://www.healio.com/ophthalmology/refractive-surgery/news/print/ocular-surgery-news/%7Bdf8c4698-b178-47f7-83cb-b3c890916b7f%7D/is-the-future-of-refractive-surgery-based-on-corneal-topography-or-wavefront. Published August 1, 2000. Accessed August 9, 2014.

30. Walsh MJ. Wavefront is showing signs of success, but can it do it alone? *Ocular Surgery News.* September 2000:41.

31. Alpins NA. Wavefront technology: a new advance that fails to answer old questions on corneal vs. refractive astigmatism correction. *J Refract Surg.* 2002;18(6):737-739.

32. Alpins N, Stamatelatos G. Clinical outcomes of laser in situ keratomileusis using combined topography and refractive wavefront treatments for myopic astigmatism. *J Cataract Refract Surg.* 2008;34(8):1250-1259.

33. Kohnen T. Reshaping the cornea: which laser profiles should we use? [editorial]. *J Cataract Refract Surg.* 2008;34(8):1225.

34. Kugler L, Cohen I, Haddad W, Wang MX. Efficacy of laser in situ keratomileusis in correcting anterior and non-anterior corneal astigmatism: comparative study. *J Cataract Refract Surg.* 2010;36(10):1745-1752.

Chapter 4

The Genesis
A Method to the Madness

FIRST, THE MADNESS

When I first began to examine astigmatism analysis and treatment to encompass laser modalities, it soon became apparent that there existed a lot of confusion about the best way to analyze and treat "the unique refractive error" of astigmatism[1,2] (Figure 4-1). Many investigators had simply compared pre- and postoperative astigmatism magnitude values alone and completely ignored any change in the astigmatic axis. Inevitably, this rendered all imperfect treatments to be "undercorrections."[3] Others calculated a mean of the axes.[4,5] None of these methods accurately assessed the success of the results nor indicated the extent to which the surgical goals were achieved. The concept of obliquely crossed cylinders was first described by Stokes[6] in 1843 and later expanded by Gartner[7] (optical decomposition) and Naylor[8] (difference in refraction due to surgery). In the 1970s, Jaffe and Clayman[9] used vector analysis to calculate the surgically induced astigmatism vector (SIA) based on corneal incisions at the 90° and 180° meridia (surgically induced refractive change using the law of cosines). Naeser's 1990 publication[10] calculated polar values of astigmatism orientation outside the 90° and 180° meridia, which was necessary to interpret the results of surgery that induced polar changes, such as cataract/intraocular lens (IOL) surgery.

The advent of refractive laser technology in the 1980s introduced the conundrum between incisional and ablation techniques, as described in Chapter 3. The pertinent question was (and is): Should the treatment be planned according to refractive cylinder values as commonly done with laser refractive surgery since its inception, or corneal astigmatism parameters as customary with incisional surgery? The overriding question for me at the time was why there should be two differing surgery paradigms to obtain essentially the same goal—reducing astigmatism to eliminate the need for spectacle correction.

Throughout the 1980s and 1990s, a multitude of approaches to astigmatism analysis and treatment had been described.[11-18] These were often contradictory and inconsistent

Alpins N. *Practical Astigmatism:
Planning and Analysis* (pp 27-31).
© 2018 SLACK Incorporated.

Sidebar 4-1
Minimizing Babel
More Than Semantics

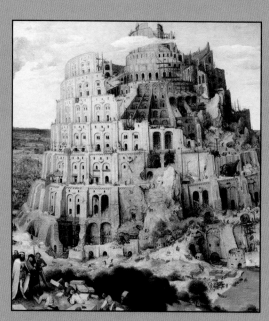

Figure 4-1. The Tower of Babel is the focus of a story in the Book of Genesis, representing the development of many languages among humankind, precipitating isolation, miscommunication, and acrimony throughout history. ("The Tower of Babel," by Pieter Bruegel the Elder, 1563.)

Standardized terminology is essential for the development and advancement of any discipline. Many terms begin with pioneers in their respective fields and become standardized by general usage. For example, Duke-Elder coined the term "residual astigmatism" to describe corneal and refractive differences[19]; Alpins introduced the term "ocular residual astigmatism" (ORA) to describe the vector difference between corneal and refractive astigmatism, and to distinguish it from the commonly used term "residual astigmatism" or astigmatism remaining after surgery.[20] The use of "residual astigmatism" to mean astigmatism remaining after surgery, in fact, conflicts with Duke-Elder's half-century-old description of a different phenomenon. The use of alternative terms such as "remaining," "resultant," or "surgical residual astigmatism" (SRA) should be considered.[21] ORA is also sometimes mistakenly called "intraocular," "lenticular," or "internal" astigmatism, which ignores the nonoptical perceptual component of the phenomenon.

Terminology is important, and is addressed frequently in this book. Perhaps, no single, more provocative obfuscation of astigmatism terminology exists than within a 2006 publication by Eydelman et al,[22] which attempted to inject its own Babel into concepts that had previously been defined in an already accepted and perfectly understandable way.[23] A more detailed description of this misadventure is contained in Chapter 20.

in application and terminology. Incisions were based on the steep corneal meridian and refractive laser surgery purely on the manifest refractive cylinder, which in many cases, did not match the corneal astigmatism in magnitude and/or orientation. To me, a better way to collect and analyze data and perform refractive procedures begged discovering. I was convinced that a systematic approach—a standardized set of guiding principles—must exist that addressed the disciplines of refractive, cataract, and corneal surgery.

THEN, THE METHOD

My introduction to refractive surgery and the need to control astigmatism began with planned extracapsular cataract extraction and IOL implantation in the early 1980s. Although emmetropia became the universal goal, the large incisions of the time—usually accompanied by suture-induced astigmatism—prevented many patients from obtaining spectacle-free vision. With a busy cataract practice, I spent almost the entirety of every Friday morning for 5 years selectively cutting sutures—two or three at a time—in patients 4 weeks after surgery. Larry Field would fit contact lenses on a sessional basis each week ay my practice. He would arrive with his manual keratometer, for which I found a great need in this suture removal process, to gauge which suture to remove next – he was truly inspirational. The process could have been called "dynamic vector analysis," since the goal of each removal session was to rotate the corneal steep meridian toward 90° as well as reduce its magnitude.

I learned much from this exercise, but realized that the scientific and mathematical evaluation of the process had a long way to go. My curiosity led me to present a paper on my results both at our lead Australian meeting in 1986 and at the Royal Hawaiian Eye Meeting in January of 1987.

I was working with my programmer, John Carragher on April 28, 1992—I remember because it was one day prior to my daughter's 21st birthday—trying to compute an analysis by corneal topographical values using refractive treatment parameters. The refractive astigmatism values used for the laser were from the manifest refraction, which still is the standard paradigm that exists now in conventional wisdom and hence the treatment parameter paradox. The corneal astigmatism uncommonly coincided with the refraction. We therefore constructed a vector diagram that satisfied his computing requirements and my outcome analysis needs by adding a crucial—but real—parameter called "target astigmatism."

In all our searches of the literature while writing my 1993 paper,[3] this "nonzero goal" had never been published as an intended refraction goal. Before long, I visualized a helpful metaphor for the Alpins Method: a golf putt (Figure 4-2). The clinical application of each of these individual "lines on a page" and others that derived from them took me 3 years of obsessive, concentrated thought to discover all the answers, the applications, and the ramifications of the prevailing unsolved conundrum of topography vs refraction. (The nonzero goal is described in greater detail in Chapter 5.) The ball got rolling with the epiphany I had that day—the eve of my daughter's 21st birthday. I knew I was onto something big. Additionally, we also had a very good birthday party that next night.

Figure 4-2. A golf putt neatly captures key features of the Alpins Method: the intended putt, or target induced astigmatism vector (TIA); the actual putt, or SIA; and the vector of a second putt that would hit the intended initial target, or the difference vector (DV).

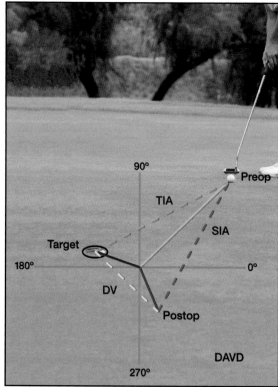

Sidebar 4-2

The Graphs That Made a Difference

Naylor's 1968 publication[8] was the first graphical representation of refractive cylinder addition on a double-angle vector diagram (DAVD). Jaffe and Clayman[9] also used DAVDs for the parallel description of corneal astigmatism analysis. In 1979, Cravy[14] showed a polar corneal analysis for cataract surgery; Naesar[10] improved on that approach in 1990 (using squared values).

All of this previous work inspired me to explain these strange new vector graphs in my first presentation at the Aspen meeting in February 1992. Still, 8 am on a good skiing day may not have been the best choice of time or audience to explain a subject I still didn't fully understand myself. But, between Aspen in February and my return home in April, in addition to working with my programmer, the "penny dropped" for me in terms of the primary concepts of the Alpins Method and its two additional vectors—the TIA and the DV. My technique used both polar diagrams and DAVDs to address corneal and refractive cylinder in any analysis.[3,20]

REFERENCES

1. Alpins N, Stamatelatos G. Chapter 24: The Cornea - Part X: Treatment and analysis of astigmatism during the laser era. In: Boyd BF, ed. *Modern Ophthalmology: The Highlights*. New Delhi, India: J.P. Medical Ltd; 2011:381-404.

2. Thornton SP. Cataract and the surgical control of astigmatism (guest editorial). *J Cataract Refract Surg*. 1989;15(1):11.

3. Alpins NA. A new method of analyzing vectors for changes in astigmatism. *J Cataract Refract Surg*. 1993;19(4):524-533.

4. Hall GW, Campion M, Sorenson CM, Monthofer S. Reduction of corneal astigmatism at cataract surgery. *J Cataract Refract Surg*. 1991;17(4):407-414.

5. Merck MP, Williams PA, Lindstrom RL. Trapezoidal keratotomy. A vector analysis. *Ophthalmology*. 1986;93(6):719-726.

6. Stokes GG. On a mode of measuring the astigmatism of a defective eye. *Transactions of the 19th meeting of the British Association for the Advancement of Science 1849*. London, England: British Association for the Advancement of Science; 1850.

7. Gartner WF. Astigmatism and optometric vectors. *Am J Optom Arch Am Acad Optom*. 1965;42:459-463.

8. Naylor EJ. Astigmatic difference in refractive errors. *Br J Ophthalmol*. 1968;52(5):422-425.

9. Jaffe NS, Clayman HM. The pathophysiology of corneal astigmatism after cataract extraction. *Transactions of the American Academy of Ophthalmology and Otolaryngology*. Rochester, MN: 1975:OP-615-OP-630.

10. Naeser K. Conversion of keratometer readings to polar values. *J Cataract Refract Surg*. 1990;16(6):741-745.

11. Axt JC. Longitudinal study of postoperative astigmatism. *J Cataract Refract Surg*. 1987;13(4):381-388.

12. Buzard KA, Laranjeira E, Fundingsland BR. Clinical results of arcuate incisions to correct astigmatism. *J Cataract Refract Surg*. 1996;22(8):1062-1069.

13. Casebeer JC. Arcuate incisions are preferable for the correction of astigmatism. *Ocular Surgery News*. August 1994:86.

14. Cravy TV. Calculation of the change in corneal astigmatism following cataract extraction. *Ophthalmic Surg*. 1979;10(1):38-49.

15. Thornton SP. *Radial and Astigmatic Keratotomy*. Thorofare, NJ: SLACK Incorporated; 1994.

16. Troutman RC, Buzard KA. *Corneal Astigmatism. Etiology, Prevention, and Management*. St Louis, MO: Mosby-Year Book; 1992.

17. Villasenor RA. Astigmatism correction: inferior incisions at risk. *Ocular Surgery News*. August 1994:80-81.

18. Waring GI. *Refractive Keratectomy for Myopia and Astigmatism*. St Louis, MO: Mosby-Year Book; 1992.

19. Duke-Elder SS. *System of Ophthalmology--Ophthalmic Optics and Refraction*. St Louis, MO: Mosby; 1970.

20. Alpins NA. New method of targeting vectors to treat astigmatism. *J Cataract Refract Surg*. 1997;23(1):65-75.

21. Alio JL, Alpins N. Excimer laser correction of astigmatism: consistent terminology for better outcomes. *J Refract Surg*. 2014;30(5):294-295.

22. Eydelman MB, Drum B, Holladay J, et al. Standardized analyses of correction of astigmatism by laser systems that reshape the cornea. *J Refract Surg*. 2006;22(1):81-95.

23. Alpins N. Terms used for the analysis of astigmatism. *J Refract Surg*. 2006;22(6):528-529.

Chapter 5

The Nonzero Target and Why It Meets Ongoing Resistance

DIFFERENCE, NO DIFFERENCE, INDIFFERENCE, OR SOMETHING ELSE?

As light travels its path to be resolved as an image by the brain, the anterior cornea is but the first influence of the human body on the organic experience of vision. Indeed, it is a critical influence, but not the only influence, and what we call astigmatism can be measured both by the shape of the anterior cornea and by the subjective sensation of vision.

This is why it is not uncommon for people to demonstrate a difference between refractive and corneal astigmatism. Empirically, I have seen this difference in many of my patients over many years of clinical practice, and have talked to colleagues around the world whose experience mirrors my own.

Although empiric observation alone is sufficient to justify many activities of medical practice, the difference between refractive and corneal astigmatism is also well supported in the literature.[1-7] Yet, some ophthalmologists appear reluctant to accept this fact, or attribute the difference to instrumentation errors or technical limitations of measurement, explanations I find unsatisfactory. Yet, other ophthalmologists appear to believe that the difference, if it exists at all, simply does not matter from the standpoint of the practicing cataract or refractive surgeon.

This type of thinking by putative leaders in the field (see Sidebar 5-1) may have contributed to any "ongoing resistance" that might exist towards the concept of ocular residual astigmatism (ORA) or other principles of the Alpins Method. Through the years, however, clinical studies and experience have confirmed the value of the Alpins Method.[2,3,6,7] My work is also the basis for "standardized analyses" of laser-based astigmatism correction published by the Astigmatism Project Group of the American National Standards Institute[8] (ANSI), which creatively altered my original terminology without reason or adequate attribution.[9,10] More on this in later chapters. If I must

Alpins N. *Practical Astigmatism:
Planning and Analysis* (pp 33-38).
© 2018 SLACK Incorporated.

Sidebar 5-1
Expert Opposition

The following comments were made in 1998 by an ophthalmologist considered to be an expert in astigmatism. Although dating back to the last gasp of the 20th century, I think echoes of these sentiments may persist in some quarters, and deserve to be addressed:

[The Alpins Method] is worthless. He's thrown away all of our traditional ways of looking at things...There is no difference between topography and refraction if you...take that surface topography [with a modern system]. He's just playing with a bunch of vectors out there.

...In the first place, you should be able to calculate exactly what it [the astigmatism] is by the surface of the cornea, and...his algorithms don't do any of that...If you don't do that, then you're correcting the problem the wrong way, because you don't know whether it's lenticular or corneal...If you don't know whether that's lenticular or corneal, why would you be using that to help correct something you did with a laser?

[If refraction and topography don't agree], it's because the topography system's analysis of those is wrong...it's because the topography system didn't center on the center of the pupil and the center of the map, and all of those things have to be fixed. You can't fix that...using a bunch of vectors, because all the topography systems are different.

Topography is the most important thing...when [topography and refraction] are different, it shows you there's something wrong with the topographic analysis.

Here in the 21st century, I find these observations almost as incomprehensible as the speaker found my publications since 1998 to be.[1,14,15,17] It is gratifying to know that vector analysis, at least, has become a standard tool in analyzing astigmatism correction in refractive surgery, and the difference between refractive and corneal astigmatism in many patients (and thus the existence of ocular residual astigmatism) continues to be measured with equipment used even today—although I've always found equipment errors and limitations to be an unlikely explanation for the clinical findings.

As for nontraditional thinking, the description probably applies to the most important medical and scientific breakthroughs in history, not to mention breakthroughs in every other area of human endeavor. I suppose I'll have to plead guilty.

find a silver lining here, it is that the ANSI authors, in 2006, were forced to write that vector analysis "is essential for evaluation of the accuracy of astigmatism treatments,"[8] a sign that any lingering general resistance to vector analysis, as perhaps seen in the 1990s, should be summarily dismissed. The Alpins Method has also been adopted as standard for reporting astigmatism results by our major journals.[11-13]

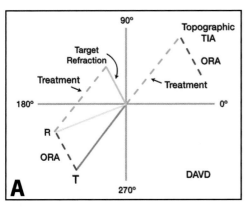

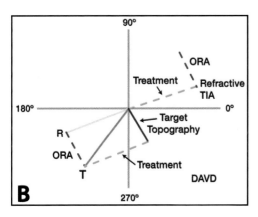

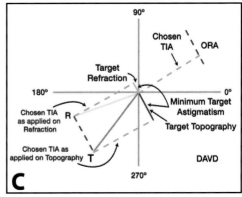

Figure 5-1. (A) These DAVDs demonstrate the treatment needed to achieve a spherical cornea by topographic (T) values; (B) the treatment needed to achieve a spherical refraction (R); (C) and a combination treatment, that nonetheless lies on the ORA vector of minimal achievable astigmatism. To achieve minimal astigmatism, the target induced astigmatism vector (TIA) must fall on the ORA.

The difference between refractive and corneal astigmatism is important because it allows the calculation of ORA and the nonzero target. Accepting that the difference exists is, thus, essential for incorporating ORA and the nonzero target into patient care. As the use of ORA and the nonzero target may contribute to improved results,[2,3,14] ignoring them can be presumed to provide less desirable results and a lower quality of patient care, no matter what "ongoing resistance" might or might not continue to exist.

AGAIN WITH THE GRAPHS

By now, the graphs in Figure 5-1 may be familiar. However, I will be asking the reader to look at them in a certain way.

Obviously, the patient who is the basis for Figure 5-1 has a difference between corneal and refractive astigmatism. As the figure legend indicates, the double-angle vector diagrams (DAVDs) illustrate the situation where astigmatism treatment is based on 100% topography (A), 100% on refraction (B), or at some intermediate point between topography and refraction (C). One can see in diagram A that, when astigmatism treatment is based solely on topography, there is—simultaneously and inescapably—a target refraction that is not zero! Similarly, if one plans treatment 100% on refraction, as shown in diagram B, there is a simultaneous and inescapable target topography that is not zero!

This is the nonzero target.

Sidebar 5-2
Birth of the Nonzero Target

Two, well-known ophthalmologists—Thomas Cravy, of Santa Maria, California, and Kristian Naeser, of Denmark—exerted a particular influence in my development of the concept of nonzero targets. Dr. Cravy brought my attention to vector analysis with a 1979 publication about astigmatism in cataract surgery, in which he used polar coordinates.[18] Dr. Naeser published a paper in 1990, where he used the square of the cosine in analyzing with-the-rule and against-the-rule astigmatism[19]; his approach improved on Euler's theorem of curved surfaces.

In examining his article, I became convinced that he was closer to the mark than Dr. Cravy, but it took me some time to digest and reconcile those two papers. By the time I returned home from the Aspen Anterior Segment Seminar meeting, in April 1992, I had the concept of the nonzero target worked out in my mind, and included it in my 1993 publication.[1]

Obviously, I owe both of these esteemed colleagues a debt of thanks for their inspiration. For the record, I met Dr. Naeser in 2006 at the European Society of Refractive and Cataract Surgeons meeting in London; we had a lunch that lasted until 6 pm—it went on and on, and we were sorry to see it end.

The common question is: Why should we care about the corneal target if we plan for and achieve the refractive target? My customary answer is that the cornea is not a spectacle lens but human tissue that the patient probably wants to use for a lifetime. Additionally, as noted in Chapter 3, in my experience, about 7% of patients have an ORA that could result in increased corneal astigmatism after laser-assisted keratomileusis (LASIK) if the treatment is based solely on refraction.[15] This cannot be a good thing, and may account for many unhappy LASIK patients, or why some patients with 20/20 postoperative visual acuity are happy and some are quite the opposite. The issue will be discussed further in the chapter on the Vector Planning approach.

In essence, a nonzero target exists in any patient who has an ORA that is not zero. What is or is not a "significant" ORA, which should be taken into consideration in surgical planning, remains a judgment call on the part of the surgeon. In my experience, an ORA of 1.00 D or greater may affect my surgical plan.[13]

A WORD OR TWO ON OPTIMAL TREATMENT

But what of the situation in graph C in Figure 5-1? What is this "intermediate treatment" all about? And so, we need to look at the figure in another way.

ORA is the vector between preoperative topography (labeled T in the figure) and preoperative refraction (labeled R in figure), and it represents the absolute minimum astigmatism that can be achieved with refractive laser surgery. The maximum correction of astigmatism is achieved when the remaining astigmatism is at its minimum and is equal to the ORA.[15,16]

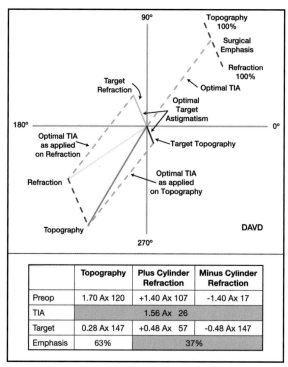

Figure 5-2. In this patient, the surgeon chooses to place 63% emphasis on the correction of topographic astigmatism and 37% emphasis on the correction of the refractive astigmatism. This "optimal treatment" (the percentage of emphasis) is determined by a linear surgical emphasis relationship described by Alpins in 1997[15]; the approach favors with-the-rule TIA.

	Topography	Plus Cylinder Refraction	Minus Cylinder Refraction
Preop	1.70 Ax 120	+1.40 Ax 107	-1.40 Ax 17
TIA		1.56 Ax 26	
Target	0.28 Ax 147	+0.48 Ax 57	-0.48 Ax 147
Emphasis	63%	37%	

Obviously, this remaining postoperative astigmatism is refractive, topographic, or a combination of both. The Alpins Method allows one to calculate the ORA as well as the parameters (laser settings) needed to eliminate 100% of T, 100% of R, or any combination of T and R equaling 100%, while leaving the absolute minimal amount of astigmatism in the eye's refractive system.[15,16]

I have described "optimal treatment," which puts more surgical emphasis on the elimination of topographic astigmatism the more unfavorably the postoperative astigmatism is expected to manifest on the cornea.[15] With this approach, the surgeon can choose which orientation he or she believes is "unfavorable." The determination of surgical emphasis, discussed in detail in my 1997 publication, remains at the discretion of the operating surgeon. Certain generally held principles, such as the notion that with-the-rule astigmatism is more desirable than against-the-rule astigmatism, less astigmatism is preferred to more astigmatism, or that advances may occur in technology or analyses that affect these choices, are taken into account. Figure 5-2 illustrates optimal treatment of a patient with typical topographic and refractive measurements, as shown in the figure's accompanying table.

In practice, in those patients we feel have "significant" ORA and who may end up with more corneal astigmatism in what we consider an "unfavorable" against-the-rule orientation, the treatment emphasis is often near the 60/40 refraction-to-topography split shown in Figure 5-2. This allocation of emphasis also seems to be a "rule of thumb" for other surgeons using the approach.

Only by understanding the nonzero target and determining refractive and topographic targets before surgery can we perform 2 essential tasks in astigmatism surgery:

1. Optimize the treatment according to the patient's individual parameters
2. Enable a valid analysis by knowing where the targets lie

Setting precise goals allows us to gauge our success, determine errors, and make various adjustments that might be needed to improve future procedures.

REFERENCES

1. Alpins NA. A new method of analyzing vectors for changes in astigmatism. *J Cataract Refract Surg.* 1993;19(4):524-533.
2. Alpins N, Stamatelatos G. Customized photoastigmatic refractive keratectomy using combined topographic and refractive data for myopia and astigmatism in eyes with forme fruste and mild keratoconus. *J Cataract Refract Surg.* 2007;33(4):591-602.
3. Alpins N, Stamatelatos G. Clinical outcomes of laser in situ keratomileusis using combined topography and refractive wavefront treatments for myopic astigmatism. *J Cataract Refract Surg.* 2008;34(8):1250-1259.
4. Frings A, Katz T, Steinberg J, Druchkiv V, Richard G, Linke SJ. Ocular residual astigmatism: effects of demographic and ocular parameters in myopic laser in situ keratomileusis. *J Cataract Refract Surg.* 2014;40(2):232-238.
5. Hashemi H, Khabazkhoob M, Peyman A, et al. The association between residual astigmatism and refractive errors in a population-based study. *J Refract Surg.* 2013;29(9):624-628.
6. Kugler L, Cohen I, Haddad W, Wang MX. Efficacy of laser in situ keratomileusis in correcting anterior and non-anterior corneal astigmatism: comparative study. *J Cataract Refract Surg.* 2010;36(10):1745-1752.
7. Qian YS, Huang J, Liu R, et al. Influence of internal optical astigmatism on the correction of myopic astigmatism by LASIK. *J Refract Surg.* 2011;27(12):863-868.
8. Eydelman MB, Drum B, Holladay J, et al. Standardized analyses of correction of astigmatism by laser systems that reshape the cornea. *J Refract Surg.* 2006;22(1):81-95.
9. Alpins N. Terms used for the analysis of astigmatism [letter]. J Refract Surg. 2006;22(6):528-529.
10. Goggin M. More on astigmatism analysis [letter]. *J Refract Surg.* 2007;23(5):430-431.
11. Author Information Pack. American Academy of Ophthalmology Web site. https://www.elsevier.com/wps/find/journaldescription.cws_home/620418?generatepdf=true. Accessed January 19, 2016.
12. Information for Authors. American Society of Cataract and Refractive Surgery Web site. http://www.jcrsjournal.org/content/authorinfo#info. Accessed September 1, 2016.
13. Reinstein DZ, Archer TJ, Randleman JB. JRS standard for reporting astigmatism outcomes of refractive surgery [editorial]. *J Refract Surg.* 2014 1;30(10):654-659.
14. Alpins NA, Tabin GC, Adams LM, Aldred GF, Kent DG, Taylor HR. Refractive versus corneal changes after photorefractive keratectomy for astigmatism. *J Refract Surg.* 1998;14(4):386-396.
15. Alpins NA. New method of targeting vectors to treat astigmatism. *J Cataract Refract Surg.* 1997;23(1):65-75.
16. Alpins NA. Corneal versus refractive astigmatism: integrated analysis. *Ocular Surgery News.* June 15, 1999:44.
17. Alpins NA. Vector analysis of astigmatism changes by flattening, steepening, and torque. *J Cataract Refract Surg.* 1997;23(10):1503-1514.
18. Cravy TV. Calculation of the change in corneal astigmatism following cataract extraction. *Ophthalmic Surg.* 1979;10(1):38-49.
19. Naeser K. Conversion of keratometer readings to polar values. *J Cataract Refract Surg.* 1990;16(6):741-745.

Chapter 6

The Basics of the Alpins Method

GETTING WITH THE PROGRAMS

A number of years ago, I published a paper titled, "Practical Astigmatism Analysis for Refractive Outcomes in Cataract and Refractive Surgery."[1] Those who use the Alpins Method quickly develop the ability to interpret the vector diagrams, values, and indices central to the methodology. Like an unfamiliar software program that soon transforms into an indispensable tool, the Alpins Method for these clinicians becomes second nature. For those who have yet to assess or utilize the method, the practicality of it may not be immediately apparent. This chapter contains an overview of the Alpins Method and a few basic observations that may help even seasoned users.

The Alpins Method is not something typically brought into the operating theater. The Alpins Method's primary applications are in planning and assessing cataract and refractive surgery. The Alpins Method is programmed into many corneal topographers using the iASSORT[2] (Alpins Statistical System for Ophthalmic Refractive surgery Techniques) software; it is also part of the comprehensive ASSORT program,[3] the VECTrAK program,[4] and online calculators for vectors,[5] femtosecond laser limbal relaxing incisions,[6] and toric intraocular lenses (IOLs).[7] These programs are detailed in Chapter 24. Briefly, ASSORT, iASSORT, and VECTrAK reveal trends that can be useful in making modifications to technique or instrumentation to improve future results. The online calculators provide Alpins Method planning and analysis of single cases at a time, whereas, the ASSORT and VECTrAK software allow analyses of multiple cases and their storage in a database.

For corneal topographers that incorporate the Alpins Method in their programming, measurements such as simulated keratometry (SimK) and axial power are automatically imported into the vector calculations. The ASSORT software is in fact a complete patient record, capable of analyzing all measurable ophthalmic parameters, such as intra-

Alpins N. *Practical Astigmatism:*
Planning and Analysis (pp 39-46).
© 2018 SLACK Incorporated.

Figure 6-1. A golf putt captures key features of the Alpins Method: the intended putt, or target induced astigmatism vector (TIA); the actual putt, or surgically induced astigmatism vector (SIA); and the vector of a second putt that would hit the intended initial target, or the difference vector (DV).

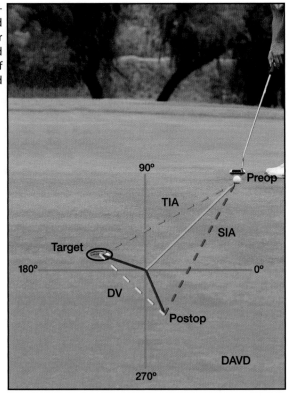

ocular pressure and glaucoma medications, visual acuities, personalized A constants, and a variety of pre- and postoperative events. Further to the analyses, the software provides for the planning of excimer laser procedures, cataract surgery including toric IOLs, and incisional surgery such as limbal relaxing incisions.

The graphical presentation of the Alpins Method includes the use of double-angle vector diagrams (DAVDs). Both polar and DAVDs are fully explored in Chapter 18. DAVDs allow calculations in a 360° sense and permit the use of rectangular (Cartesian) coordinates. References at the end of this chapter[1,8-11] detail the trigonometry involved for the interested reader.

THE THREE FUNDAMENTAL VECTORS

Vectors are mathematical expressions having both magnitude and direction. Vectors cannot be measured, but only calculated. Astigmatism, which can be measured—with cylinder power and axis (refractive) or magnitude and meridian (corneal)—is ideally suited for vector analysis.

Three fundamental vectors of the Alpins Method are neatly captured by an analogy to a golf putt (Figure 6-1). As golfers know, putting the ball into the cup on a flat green is simple to envision, but not always easy to accomplish. The putt in this case is a vector of the astigmatic treatment (TIA), possessing both magnitude (length) and direction (axis of the vector). When the putt misses the target cup, one of two possible events have

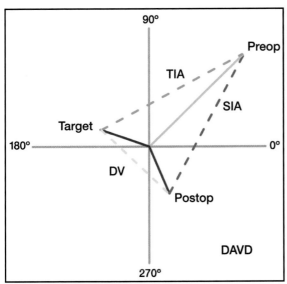

Figure 6-2. The TIA, SIA, and DV are analogous to the golf putt shown in Figure 6-1. The TIA, SIA, and DV are calculated from (1) the patient's preoperative astigmatism; (2) the targeted astigmatism the surgeon plans to achieve; and (3) the actual achieved effect of the surgery.

occurred: the force with which the ball was struck was either too great or too soft, or the direction in which it was hit was either clockwise or counterclockwise to that required. A combination of the two is most common. The single most revealing parameter of the overall success of a putt is the length required for a second putt to place the ball in the cup.

At its most basic, the Alpins Method is no more complicated than this golf analogy. The intended effect of the astigmatism surgery (the path from the ball to the cup) is the TIA.[1,9] The actual putt (the path the ball takes when hit) corresponds to the SIA.[12] The second putt needed to hit the cup corresponds to the DV, or the amount and orientation of the astigmatism treatment required to achieve the original target. A DAVD of these three fundamental vectors is shown in Figure 6-2, and comprises the essence of the Alpins Method. (Note—In clinical practice, the calculated DV is not used to plan a secondary procedure, if one becomes necessary. Instead, new calculations are made based on the patient's existing refractive and corneal measurements, and a new plan is created as if it were a primary procedure.)

REVEALING RELATIONSHIPS

The various relationships between the SIA and TIA indicate whether treatment was on axis or off axis, whether too much or too little treatment was applied and the adjustment that would be necessary if one had the chance to perform the same astigmatic correction again from the start. The TIA quantifies intended treatment at the corneal plane and is key to allowing an integrated analysis to be performed by any modality of astigmatism measurement—corneal or refractive. (Note—To achieve a valid analysis with the Alpins Method, all refractive astigmatism values are converted to the corneal plane.[10,11,13-16])

The TIA, SIA, and DV allow the calculation of a variety of helpful indices,[1,9-11] which are described in detail in Chapter 7:

- **Correction index (CI)**—What the surgery actually induced vs what the surgery was meant to induce. The CI is preferably 1.0; it is > 1.0 if an overcorrection of astigmatism occurs and < 1.0 if there is an undercorrection of astigmatism.
- **Coefficient of adjustment (CA)**—The inverse of the CI, the CA quantifies the modification needed to the initial surgery plan to have achieved a CI of 1.0. The CA can be used to refine nomograms for future procedures.
- **Magnitude of error (ME)**—The arithmetic difference between the magnitudes of the SIA and the TIA. It is positive for overcorrections and negative for undercorrections of astigmatism.
- **Angle of error (AE)**—The angle described by the vectors of the intended correction vs the achieved correction (SIA minus TIA). The AE is positive if the achieved correction is on an axis counterclockwise to where it was intended and negative if the achieved correction is clockwise to its intended axis.
- **Index of success (IOS)**—The IOS is a relative measure of success. The IOS is a measure of the relative effectiveness of various surgical procedures and is preferably zero.
- **Flattening effect (FE)**—The amount of astigmatism reduction achieved at the intended treatment meridian; that is, the effective portion of the SIA (FE = SIA cos2.AE).
- **Flattening index (FI)**—The FI is calculated by dividing the FE by the TIA and is preferably 1.0.

These indices can be subjected to conventional forms of statistical analysis, generating averages, means, standard deviations, etc, for each individual component of surgery.

SURGICAL EMPHASIS AND OPTIMAL TREATMENT

Ocular residual astigmatism (ORA), further described in Chapters 5 and 9, is the vector between preoperative corneal astigmatism as measured, for example, by topography (T) and preoperative refractive cylinder (R), and it represents the absolute minimum of astigmatism that can be achieved surgically in the eye (Figure 6-3). The maximum correction of astigmatism is achieved when the remaining astigmatism is at its minimum and is equal to the ORA.[10,17]

ORA exists in any eye in which refractive and corneal astigmatism are of unequal magnitude and/or axis. In a study of 100 consecutive eyes,[10] I found that the magnitude of topographic astigmatism exceeded refractive astigmatism in 59 patients; refractive astigmatism was greater in the remaining 41. A minority of patients had < 10° of angular separation between topographic and refractive measurements; many had 10° or greater separation (up to almost 80°). Interestingly, for patients with topographical steep meridia closer to 90°, the magnitude of topographical astigmatism exceeded that of refractive astigmatism; and for those with topographical steep meridia closer to 180°, refractive astigmatism had the greater value. This finding supports the widely-held idea that people have a greater optical tolerance for with-the-rule corneal astigmatism.

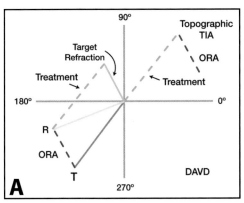

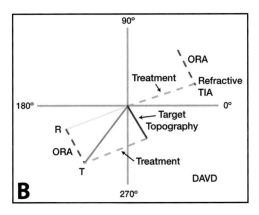

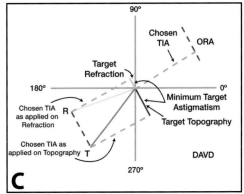

Figure 6-3. (A) These DAVDs demonstrate the treatment needed to achieve a spherical cornea by topographic (T) values; (B) the treatment needed to achieve a spherical refraction (R); and (C) a combination treatment, that nonetheless terminates on the ORA vector of minimal achievable astigmatism. To achieve minimal astigmatism, the TIA must end on the ORA.

Sidebar 6-1

The Common Question
Why Not Use Refraction as the Only Treatment Parameter?

The question dates back to the original publication[9] of the Alpins Method in 1993: Why not use refraction as the only treatment parameter for both cylinder and sphere? The penalty for sculpting the spectacle astigmatism onto the cornea is that all ORA would remain as surgical residual astigmatism (SRA) on the cornea. This is contrary to established principles of corneal surgery. In my experience, about 7% of patients have an ORA that could result in increased corneal astigmatism after laser-assisted in situ keratomileusis if the target is based solely on refraction.[10]

The cornea is not a spectacle lens but human tissue. The potential exists for increased spherical aberrations and coma with degradation of the perceived image.[18] The eye's optical system, independent of spectacle correction, will continue to depend on optimal astigmatic correction by the shape of the anterior corneal surface.

Ignoring the nonzero target for corneal astigmatism, an unavoidable byproduct of treating only the refractive error, may account for many unhappy LASIK patients with or without 20/20 visual acuity caused by the excess corneal astigmatism remaining where the ORA is significant.

Enter the concept of "optimal treatment." The Alpins Method allows one to calculate the ORA, as well as the parameters (laser settings) needed to eliminate 100% of T, 100% of R, or any combination of T and R equaling 100%, which leaves the absolute minimal amount of astigmatism in the eye's refractive system and its optical correction.[10,17] The Alpins Method also calculates an "optimal treatment," which puts more surgical emphasis on the elimination of topographic astigmatism the more unfavorably the postoperative astigmatism is expected to reside on the cornea[10] (Figure 6-4).

The surgical emphasis of the treatment shown in Figure 6-4 is the position of the chosen TIA relative to topographic and refractive TIAs, and is expressed as a percentage. The maximum correction is possible when the surgical emphasis line overlies the ORA line connecting the ends of the topographic and refractive TIAs, and when the selected TIA terminates where it intersects this line. Surgical emphasis determines how the astigmatism that unavoidably remains (ie, the ORA) will be distributed.

With optimal treatment, the target falls parallel to the ORA line, of course, and with this approach, the surgeon can choose which orientation he or she believes is favorable or unfavorable. The determination of surgical emphasis remains at the discretion of the operating surgeon. Figure 6-4 illustrates optimal treatment of a patient with typical topographic and refractive measurements, and is based on the widespread observation that with-the-rule astigmatism is favorable and against-the-rule astigmatism is unfavorable. Further investigation of the effect of astigmatism orientation—oblique astigmatism, for example—could significantly add to our knowledge of astigmatism planning, analysis, and treatment, as well as to patient informed consent.

The optimal treatment of astigmatism is thus achieved, not only when the sum of the topographic and refractive astigmatism equals the minimum target value achievable for that eye, but also when the remaining astigmatism is appropriately apportioned to topography and refraction according to the orientation of the target astigmatism. The optimal treatment of astigmatism seeks to achieve less corneal astigmatism than if treating by refraction alone, with an attempt to influence its orientation favorably by adjusting the magnitude of the corneal target.

A BASE FOR MOVING FORWARD

The basics of the Alpins Method create a foundation for understanding other important concepts described in this book: the Vector Planning approach, topographic disparity, corneal topographic astigmatism, refractive surprises after toric IOL implantation, and more. Despite the insight and utility that many practitioners derive from the Alpins Method and its related tools, the growing use of the method depends greatly on its clinical practicality.

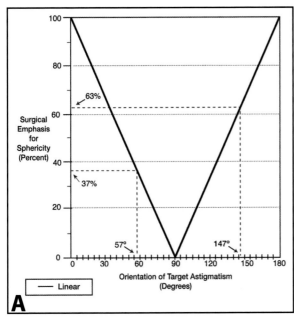

A

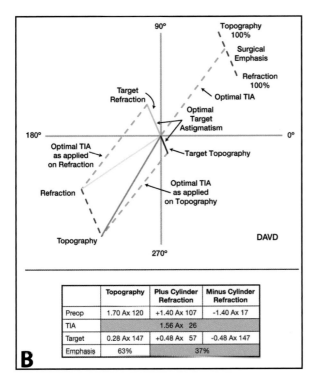

B

Figure 6-4. The Alpins Method calculates "optimal treatment" based on the linear relationship shown in graph A. Future research may determine that the actual relationship is nonlinear or otherwise varies from the graph shown. In this example, the meridian of target topography is 147° which lies 57° from a with-the-rule orientation of 90°. Using this linear relationship, the surgeon may decide to apportion 57° of 90° (63.3%) emphasis to a topography-based goal of zero astigmatism (147° intersects the linear emphasis line at 63%). This results in a 37% emphasis on the correction of refractive astigmatism. Graph B is a DAVD of the optimal TIA and treatment parameters.

REFERENCES

1. Alpins NA, Goggin M. Practical astigmatism analysis for refractive outcomes in cataract and refractive surgery. *Surv Ophthalmol.* 2004;49(1):109-122.

2. About iASSORT. ASSORT Web site. http://www.assort.com/products/iassort. Accessed September 29, 2014.

3. ASSORT Web site. http://www.assort.com. Accessed April 22, 2014.

4. About VECTrAK. ASSORT Web site. http://www.assort.com/assort.asp?id=2. Accessed September 29, 2014.

5. ASSORT Vector Calculator. ASSORT Web site. http://www.assort.com/ASSORT-vector-calculator-intro.asp. Accessed September 29, 2014.

6. Femto LRI Calculator. ASSORT Web site. http://www.assort.com/ASSORT-femto-calculator-intro.asp. Accessed September 29, 2014.

7. ASSORT Toric IOL Calculator. ASSORT Web site. http://www.assort.com/ASSORT-toric-calculator-intro.asp. Accessed February 18. 2014.

8. Alpins N, Stamatelatos G. Chapter 24: The Cornea - Part X: Treatment and analysis of astigmatism during the laser era. In: Boyd BF, ed. *Modern Ophthalmology: The Highlights.* New Delhi, India: J.P. Medical Ltd; 2010:381-404.

9. Alpins NA. A new method of analyzing vectors for changes in astigmatism. *J Cataract Refract Surg.* 1993;19(4):524-533.

10. Alpins NA. New method of targeting vectors to treat astigmatism. *J Cataract Refract Surg.* 1997;23(1):65-75.

11. Alpins NA. Vector analysis of astigmatism changes by flattening, steepening, and torque. *J Cataract Refract Surg.* 1997;23(10):1503-1514.

12. Jaffe NS, Clayman HM. The pathophysiology of corneal astigmatism after cataract extraction. *Transactions of the American Academy of Ophthalmology and Otolaryngology.* Rochester, MN: 1975:OP-615-OP-630.

13. Alpins NA, Tabin GC, Adams LM, Aldred GF, Kent DG, Taylor HR. Refractive versus corneal changes after photorefractive keratectomy for astigmatism. *J Refract Surg.* 1998;14(4):386-396.

14. Goggin M, Pesudovs K. Assessment of surgically induced astigmatism: toward an international standard. *J Cataract Refract Surg.* 1998;24(12):1548-1550.

15. Holladay JT, Dudeja DR, Koch DD. Evaluating and reporting astigmatism for individual and aggregate data. *J Cataract Refract Surg.* 1998;24(1):57-65.

16. Weiss RA, Berke W, Gottlieb L, Horvath P. Clinical importance of accurate refractor vertex distance measurements prior to refractive surgery. *J Refract Surg.* 2002;18(4):444-448.

17. Alpins NA. Corneal versus refractive astigmatism: integrated analysis. *Ocular Surgery News.* June 15, 1999:44.

18. Seiler T, Reckmann W, Maloney RK. Effective spherical aberration of the cornea as a quantitative descriptor in corneal topography. *J Cataract Refract Surg.* 1993;19(suppl):155-165.

Chapter 7

The Astigmatic Indices
Useful Measures That Make It All Worthwhile

THIS MEANS WAR

General William Tecumseh Sherman once noted that "War is hell." A continent and four score years away, Winston Churchill posited that "History is written by the victors." In ophthalmology, my experience has been that new and useful concepts utilizing well-crafted terminology may have to dig in and do battle for a couple of decades before becoming an accepted standard.

And now for a little history. The Alpins Method has acquired many allies over the years. Well over 1000 papers in the literature have referenced my publications. Journal editors have acclaimed or endorsed the approach.[1-6] Remarking on a study by Borasio et al,[7] an editorial[4] in the *Journal of Cataract & Refractive Surgery* (*JCRS*) noted that:

> …[t]he Borasio paper demonstrates the elegance and usefulness of the Alpins method. It is gratifying to see that several elements of Alpins' approach have been incorporated into the recommendations of the Astigmatism Project Group of the American National Standards Institute,[8] although I believe that Alpins' work was not acknowledged as fully as was warranted. In addition, Eydelman et al[8] changed Alpins' terminology, raising the concern that this will create confusion in the literature.

An editorial in the same journal by a different editor two years later[5] was titled "Impact of Citation Practices: Beyond Journal Impact Factors," and contained this passage:

> …omission of key references or attribution of work to a secondary reference rather than a primary source can distort the field by re-mapping key contributions inaccurately. This challenging issue, a recently noted example of which is Alpins'[9] under-acknowledged vector approach to analyzing surgically induced

Alpins N. *Practical Astigmatism:*
Planning and Analysis (pp 47-54).
© 2018 SLACK Incorporated.

astigmatism, can be addressed through errata and correspondences[4]; but once in the literature, such errors are prone to propagation. Errors of omission or inaccurate attribution also occur when review articles are used in lieu of primary sources...

MAKE-UP TEXT

Table 7-1 appeared in a 2014 editorial by Reinstein et al[10] in the *Journal of Refractive Surgery* (*JRS*). The editorial, which describes the journal's new standard for reporting astigmatism results, refers to a paper by Eydelman et al,[8] published previously in that journal and representing the efforts of a committee of the American National Standards Institute (ANSI). The editorial by Reinstein et al[10] notes:

> The majority of the astigmatism analysis methods included in the ANSI article were directly adapted from the methods developed and originally published by Alpins in 1993,[9,11,12] in many instances with simple renaming of the original terminology. Although this was highlighted at the time in correspondence to the Editor,[13] the altered terminology has been used subsequently in many publications reporting astigmatism...[14] Our position at the Journal is that all future reports of astigmatism should adhere to the original terminology as described by Alpins.[9,11,12]

The editor of the journal—in reply to my letter[13] pointing out the "simple renaming" of my original terminology in the article by Eydelman et al[8]—held that the ANSI article "does not qualify for peer review, as it is a completed formal document from ANSI and is published as the project group's report." I was surprised by this response. In any event, this "simple renaming" of the concepts and terminology I had previously developed[9,15,16] went from manuscript to printed page, apparently unchallenged and unedited.

Reinstein et al[10] pointed out that the ANSI terminology has been picked up by many authors, compounding the confusion. The editorial by Reinstein et al and establishing a standard for reporting astigmatism results both went far in eliminating that confusion, and amounted to a vindication of the Alpins Method—after more than two decades. However, as you will see in the chapters ahead, terminology and reference mistakes continued to be made in the years since the *JRS* editorial, and efforts continue in attempting to correct them.

THE INDICES OF THE ALPINS METHOD

The target induced astigmatism vector (TIA), surgically induced astigmatism vector (SIA), and the difference vector (DV), and the description and calculation of their various relationships (the indices), comprise the essence of the Alpins Method.[9,11,12,15,16] Figure 7-1 shows the standard charts now mandated by the *JRS* for articles reporting astigmatism results[10]; the charts are based on the Alpins Method.

Drawing inspiration from many people and events around me over the years (Sidebar 7-1), I have described the following indices, all of which are neatly summarized in a 2004 publication[15] in *Survey of Ophthalmology*:

Table 7-1
Terminology for Reporting Astigmatism

Alpins Method	ANSI	Reason
Target induced astigmatism vector (TIA)	Intended refractive correction	TIA is easily understood as the astigmatic correction that was attempted. On the other hand, the term "intended refractive correction" could also be interpreted as inclusive of sphere (eg as spherical equivalent).
Surgically induced astigmatism vector (SIA)	Surgically induced refractive correction (SIRC)	SIRC does not specifically apply to astigmatism (it can be misinterpreted as inclusive of sphere), whereas SIA can only be interpreted as the astigmatism achieved by the surgery. Also, SIA is a term that can be applied to either manifest refractive or corneal analysis, whereas SIRC would be inappropriate for corneal analysis alone.
Magnitude of error	Error of magnitude	This describes the arithmetic difference between the SIA and TIA (ie, the magnitude of the error). The term "error of magnitude" implies that the error is related to the magnitude of the treatment, which is not necessarily the case.
Angle of error	Error of angle	This describes the angle between the axis of the SIA and the axis of the TIA (ie, it is the angle of the error between these two vectors). It is not an error of an angle because by definition there are no angles in astigmatism (only axes); an angle does not specify a position in space, whereas an axis specifies the actual orientation.
Difference vector (DV)	Error vector	This is literally defined as the vectorial "difference" between the TIA and SIA vectors; this difference may not represent an "error" in the surgery or treatment because other factors could be in play causing such a "difference" to occur. In addition, the Alpins Method has precedence with no added benefit to changing the terminology.
Correction index	Correction ratio	This is defined as the SIA divided by the TIA. Although this could be described as either a ratio or an index, the Alpins Method has precedence with no added benefit to changing the terminology.
Index of success	Error ratio	This is defined as the DV divided by the TIA and provides the surgeon with a measure of the "success" in correcting the astigmatism rather than introducing the negative connotation of "error." In addition, the Alpins Method has precedence with no added benefit to changing the terminology.

Abbreviation: ANSI; American National Standards Institute.

A 2014 editorial in the *Journal of Refractive Surgery* outlined the journal's new standard in reporting astigmatism results. The new standard uses Alpins' original terminology[9, 11, 17] as opposed to terminology proposed by a committee of the American National Standard Institute (ANSI).[8] The definitions of the ANSI terms show them to be identical to those set out by Alpins previously. Reprinted with permission from Reinstein DZ, Archer TJ, Randleman JB. JRS standard for reporting astigmatism outcomes of refractive surgery [editorial]. *J Refract Surg*. 2014;30(10):654-659.

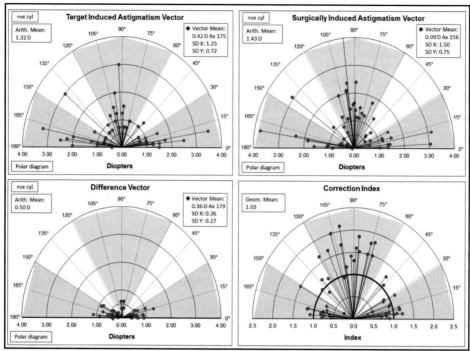

Figure 7-1. This figure, from an editorial by Reinstein et al,[10] establishes the standard graphs the *Journal of Refractive Surgery* will require for reporting the outcomes of astigmatism correction. Based on the Alpins Method, the graphs show the TIA, SIA, DV, and CI. This standard of reporting was subsequently adopted by *Ophthalmology* and *JCRS*.[17,18] (Reprinted with permission from Reinstein DZ, Archer TJ, Randleman JB. JRS standard for reporting astigmatism outcomes of refractive surgery [editorial]. *J Refract Surg*. 2014;30(10):654-659.)

Analysis of Treatment

1. TIA: The astigmatic change (by magnitude and axis) the surgery was intended to induce.[9]

2. SIA: The amount and axis of astigmatic change the surgery actually induces.

   Correction index (CI): Calculated by determining the ratio of the SIA to the TIA (what the surgery actually induces versus what the surgery was meant to induce), calculated by dividing SIA (actual effect) by TIA (target effect). The CI is preferably 1.0 (it is greater than 1.0 if an overcorrection occurs and less than 1.0 if there is an undercorrection).[17]

   Magnitude of error (ME): The arithmetic difference between the magnitudes of the SIA and TIA. The magnitude of error is positive for overcorrections and negative for undercorrections.

   Angle of error (AE): The angle described by the vectors of the achieved correction versus the intended correction. The AE is positive if the achieved correction is on an axis counterclockwise (CCW) to its intended axis and negative if the achieved correction is clockwise (CW) to its intended axis.[9]

3. DV: The change (by magnitude and axis) that would enable the initial surgery to achieve the original target on the second attempt. The DV is an absolute measure of success and is preferably 0.[9]

> *Index of Success (IOS)*: Calculated by dividing the DV by the TIA (the intended treatment). The IOS is a relative measure of success and is preferably 0.

4. Flattening effect (FE): The amount of astigmatism reduction achieved by the effective proportion of the SIA at the intended meridian. (FE = SIACos2 × AE).

> *Flattening Index (FI)*: Calculated by dividing the FE by the TIA and is preferably 1.0.[12]

5. Torque: The amount of astigmatic change induced by the SIA that has been ineffective in reducing astigmatism at the intended meridian but has caused rotation and a small increase in the existing astigmatism. Torque lies 45° CCW to the SIA if positive and 45° CW to the SIA if negative.[9]

6. Nomogram calculator for astigmatism: An additional parameter is available from [t]his method of astigmatism analysis that enables the achievement of a full correction of astigmatism magnitude in future treatments based on past experience. This is:

> *Coefficient of adjustment (CA)*: (derived by dividing TIA by SIA, the CI inverse), to adjust future astigmatism treatment (TIA) magnitude. Its value is preferably 1.0.[9]

Analysis of Ocular Status

1. Ocular residual astigmatism (ORA): A vectorial measure of the non-corneal component of total refractive astigmatism, that is, the vector difference between refractive and corneal astigmatism calculated in diopters.[19]

2. Topographic disparity (TD): A vectorial measure of irregular astigmatism calculated in diopters.[20] The greater the TD the more irregular the cornea.

Analogous Parameters for Parallel Comparisons of Spherical Change at Corneal Plane[11,21]

1. Spherical correction index (S.CI):

> <u>Spherical equivalent correction achieved</u>
>
> Spherical equivalent correction targeted

2. Spherical difference (SDiff):

> [Spherical equivalent achieved—spherical equivalent targeted] (absolute)

3. Index of success of spherical change (S.IOS):

   <u>Spherical difference</u>

   Spherical equivalent correction targeted

4. To express indices as percentages:

   Percentage of astigmatism corrected: CI × 100

   Percentage of astigmatism reduction at the intended axis: FI × 100

   Percentage success of astigmatism surgery: (1.0 − IOS) × 100

   Percentage of sphere corrected: SCI × 100

   Percentage success of spherical surgery: (1.0 − Sph IOS) × 100

It should be noted that SIA was described by Stokes[22] and Jaffe and Clayman[23] before my 1993 publication.[9] Unlike prior approaches to astigmatism analysis, the indices of the Alpins Method[9,11,12,15,16] can be subjected to conventional forms of statistical analysis, generating averages, means, standard deviations, etc, for each individual component of surgery. The Alpins Method comprehensively addresses the outcome analysis requirements of the entire cornea and the eye's refractive correction for the purpose of examining success in cataract and refractive surgery. The Alpins Method also can be applied separately to the two hemimeridians of the cornea, allowing advanced astigmatism analysis for patients with irregular astigmatism.

The war may or may not be over, depending on how influential and convincing the new reporting standards of *JCRS, JRS,* and *Ophthalmology* are. The field as a whole will make the final call. And at least for the time being, the history lesson is over.

Sidebar 7-1
Inspiration All Around Me

The Alpins Method indices came together over a period of 4 or 5 years. I was absorbed in this world for the entire period, testing the patience of my wife and family and probably many others. It proved to be a significant challenge for me; it was a comprehensive methodology that did not fall easily into place. I empathize with those who struggle with it, although, like any discipline, it gets much easier with practice. My 3 pivotal papers were published in 1993[9] and 1997.[12,17] A fourth paper, on irregular astigmatism, was published in 1998.[18]

Early on, I was referred to a computer programmer named John Carragher. John had a background in engineering often requiring the construction of tunnels for mines in Western Australia. Tunnels often were dug through mountains; engineers would start digging on both sides of a mountain at the same time and would have to meet perfectly in the middle. It was a vector calculation in three dimensions, and a perfect grounding for vectorial analysis. John would ask me questions that I hadn't considered, and I would go home and work it out. The back and forth resulted in the ASSORT (Alpins Statistical System for Ophthalmic Refractive surgery Techniques) program.

A patent attorney also inspired new ideas. He would create sketches as part of the patent process; although he didn't understand what they meant, I quickly saw their potential. My countryman and colleague Hugh Taylor was a reviewer for one of my 1997 papers,[17] and his comments were very helpful to me. Papers by Cravy[24] and Naeser[25] inspired me to develop a technique for refractive surgery requiring the concept of a nonzero target (Chapter 5).

My mentor in astigmatism correction was Spencer Thornton, of Nashville, Tennessee. I met Spencer at the Royal Hawaiian Eye Meeting in 1986, and he was the first person to invite me to be a speaker at an international ophthalmology meeting. Spencer encouraged me, visited my home in Melbourne, and became a solid friend.

Geoff Tabin, now of Park City, Utah, is an extraordinary man. He is a cofounder of the Himalayan Cataract Project and is one of only four individuals to climb the highest peaks on all seven continents. Geoff is a professor of ophthalmology and visual sciences and codirector of the Outreach Division at the John A. Moran Eye Center and University of Utah, Salt Lake City. Geoff helped me write my first book chapter during his fellowship in Hugh Taylor's Melbourne University Department of Ophthalmology in 1993 and 1994, in a book by McGhee and coeditors.[26] I was tagged to write the chapter, and introduced to Geoff, by my friend and coeditor of the book, Hugh Taylor.

The people who inspired me, in fact, are exceedingly numerous. I can only hope that the major ones are credited somewhere in this book, and if I overlook anyone, I humbly apologize.

REFERENCES

1. Koch DD. Excimer laser technology: new options coming to fruition [editorial]. *J Cataract Refract Surg.* 1997;23(10):1429-1430.

2. Koch DD. Reporting astigmatism data [editorial]. *J Cataract Refract Surg.* 1998;24(12):1545.

3. Koch DD. How should we analyze astigmatic data? [editorial]. *J Cataract Refract Surg.* 2001;27(1):1-3.

4. Koch DD. Astigmatism analysis: the spectrum of approaches [editorial]. *J Cataract Refract Surg.* 2006;32(12):1977-1978.

5. Dupps WJ, Jr. Impact of citation practices: beyond journal impact factors [editorial]. *J Cataract Refract Surg.* 2008;34(9):1419-1421.

6. Kohnen T. Reshaping the cornea: which laser profiles should we use? [editorial]. *J Cataract Refract Surg.* 2008;34(8):1225.

7. Borasio E, Mehta JS, Maurino V. Torque and flattening effects of clear corneal temporal and on-axis incisions for phacoemulsification. *J Cataract Refract Surg.* 2006;32(12):2030-2038.

8. Eydelman MB, Drum B, Holladay J, et al. Standardized analyses of correction of astigmatism by laser systems that reshape the cornea. *J Refract Surg.* 2006;22(1):81-95.

9. Alpins NA. A new method of analyzing vectors for changes in astigmatism. *J Cataract Refract Surg.* 1993;19(4):524-533.

10. Reinstein DZ, Archer TJ, Randleman JB. JRS standard for reporting astigmatism outcomes of refractive surgery [editorial]. *J Refract Surg.* 2014;30(10):654-659.

11. Alpins N. Astigmatism analysis by the Alpins method. *J Cataract Refract Surg.* 2001;27(1):31-49.

12. Alpins NA. Vector analysis of astigmatism changes by flattening, steepening, and torque. *J Cataract Refract Surg.* 1997;23(10):1503-1514.

13. Alpins N. Terms used for the analysis of astigmatism [letter]. *J Refract Surg.* 2006;22(6):528-529.

14. Alpins N. Vector analysis with the femtosecond laser [letter]. *J Cataract Refract Surg.* 2014;40(7):1246-1247.

15. Alpins NA, Goggin M. Practical astigmatism analysis for refractive outcomes in cataract and refractive surgery. *Surv Ophthalmol.* 2004;49(1):109-122.

16. Alpins N, Stamatelatos G. Chapter 24: The Cornea - Part X: Treatment and analysis of astigmatism during the laser era. In: Boyd BF, ed. *Modern Ophthalmology: The Highlights.* New Delhi, India: J.P. Medical Ltd; 2010:381-404.

17. Author Information Pack. American Academy of Ophthalmology Web site. https://www.elsevier.com/wps/find/journaldescription.cws_home/620418?generatepdf=true. Accessed January 19, 2016.

18. Information for Authors. American Society of Cataract and Refractive Surgery Web site. http://www.jcrsjournal.org/content/authorinfo#info. Accessed September 1, 2016.

19. Alpins NA. New method of targeting vectors to treat astigmatism. *J Cataract Refract Surg.* 1997;23(1):65-75.

20. Alpins NA. Treatment of irregular astigmatism. *J Cataract Refract Surg.* 1998;24(5):634-646.

21. Alpins NA, Tabin GC, Adams LM, Aldred GF, Kent DG, Taylor HR. Refractive versus corneal changes after photorefractive keratectomy for astigmatism. *J Refract Surg.* 1998;14(4):386-396.

22. Stokes GG. On a mode of measuring the astigmatism of a defective eye. *Transactions of the 19th meeting of the British Association for the Advancement of Science 1849.* London, England: British Association for the Advancement of Science; 1850.

23. Jaffe NS, Clayman HM. The pathophysiology of corneal astigmatism after cataract extraction. *Transactions of the American Academy of Ophthalmology and Otolaryngology.* Rochester, MN: 1975:OP-615-OP-630.

24. Cravy TV. Calculation of the change in corneal astigmatism following cataract extraction. *Ophthalmic Surg.* 1979;10(1):38-49.

25. Naeser K. Conversion of keratometer readings to polar values. *J Cataract Refract Surg.* 1990;16(6):741-745.

26. Alpins NA, Tabin GC, Taylor HR. Photoastigmatic refractive keratectomy (PARK). In: McGhee C, Taylor HR, Garty DS, Trokel SL, eds. *Excimer Lasers in Ophthalmology.* London, England: Martin Dunitz; 1997:243-259.

Chapter 8

The Flattening, Steepening, and Rotation of Astigmatism

A Brief Visit With the Vector Planning Approach

A substantial portion of this book describes concepts I have developed that allow for the use of vectors in planning, treating, and analyzing cataract/incisional and refractive surgery.[1-5] Many of the combined elements of this approach are collectively called the *Vector Planning* approach and are described in greater detail in Chapter 13. The full armamentarium of the Vector Planning approach, including the use of the generated indices of astigmatism analysis (Chapter 7), collectively comprise the Alpins Method. This chapter concerns the use of the Alpins Method to understand flattening, steepening, and torque, or rotation of astigmatism. I defined these concepts and their analysis initially in 1997[4]; together with other applications of the Alpins Method, they are also discussed in a 1999 series of articles in *Ocular Surgery News*.[6-10] As with other terminology of the Alpins Method, the terms flattening, steepening, and torque have occasionally been altered or misapplied[11] in the succeeding years. The adoption of the Alpins Method terminology and graphic presentation by the major journals should ameliorate the situation over time.[12-16]

The *Ocular Surgery News* series[6-10] is notable since it addresses, in succession and in basic terms, the following:

1. Vector analysis and mapping
2. Flattening, steepening, and torque
3. The integrated analysis of corneal and refractive astigmatism
4. The treatment of irregular astigmatism
5. A useful new measure of irregular astigmatism, called topographic disparity

This book contains chapters devoted to all these topics.

By way of a brief review, necessary to understand the slightly more complex question of flattening, steepening, and torque, we recall that three fundamental vectors of the Alpins Method are neatly captured by an analogy to a golf putt (Figure 8-1). The

Alpins N. *Practical Astigmatism: Planning and Analysis* (pp 55-63).
© 2018 SLACK Incorporated.

Figure 8-1. A golf putt captures key features of the Alpins Method: the intended putt, or TIA; the actual putt, or SIA; and the vector of a second putt that would hit the intended initial target, or the DV.

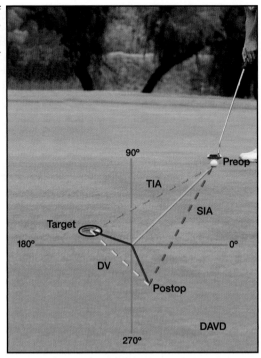

Figure 8-2. Vector mapping of the golf putt shown in Figure 8-1 demonstrates some fundamentals of the Alpins Method.

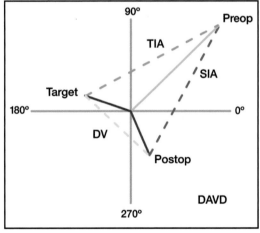

targeted initial putt is the target induced astigmatism vector (TIA), which is the astigmatic change, by magnitude and axis, which the surgeon intends to induce in order to correct the patient's preexisting astigmatism. The actual putt (the path the ball follows when hit) corresponds to the surgically induced astigmatism vector (SIA), which is the amount and axis of astigmatic change the surgeon actually induces with the procedure. If the golfer misses the cup, the difference vector (DV) corresponds to the second putt; that is, a putt that would allow the golfer to hit the cup with the ball on the second attempt, thus, providing one parameter of astigmatism surgery that effectively measures the error (by magnitude and axis). Figure 8-2 is the basic graphical representation of the golf putt in Figure 8-1.

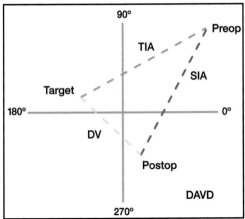

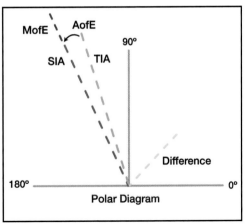

Figure 8-3. The TIA, SIA and DV are calculated from joining (1) the patient's preoperative astigmatism; (2) the targeted astigmatism the surgeon plans to achieve; and (3) the actual achieved effect of the surgery in this double-angle vector diagram. The dashed lines joined by the ends of these measurements are the vectors for SIA, TIA, and DV.

Figure 8-4. Depicting vectors in a 180° polar sense reflects the actual surgical vectors—that is, the actual axes as superimposed over the eye. The relative lengths of the vectors correspond to dioptric measurements.

POLAR AND DOUBLE-ANGLE VECTOR DIAGRAMS

Figures 8-3 and 8-4 are like cousins that need to be understood both together and separately. Figure 8-3 is a double-angle vector diagram (DAVD), which allows calculations in a 360° sense and permits the use of rectangular coordinates. DAVDs are a simple mathematical construct that allow for the calculation of vectors by adding and subtracting astigmatisms; they do not have any clinical significance. Figure 8-4 depicts the polar coordinates of the same case as shown in Figures 8-3. The polar coordinates illustrate the situation in a 180° sense; these coordinates represent the surgical vectors. The surgical vectors are directly related to the various meridia as they would appear superimposed over the eye. The length of the vectors represents the dioptric arithmetic values; the angles and magnitudes of error are the respective differences between axis and magnitude of the SIA and TIA. The mathematics underlying these graphs is detailed in the original published paper.[2]

In the Alpins Method, it's important to remember that vectors represent the amount of steepening occurring at that orientation. Also, vectors differ in their properties from astigmatism in that they can only be calculated, not measured like astigmatism. This distinction is important, as confusion can arise because vectors share the same units—diopters and degrees.

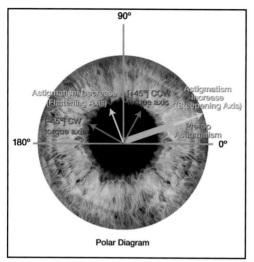

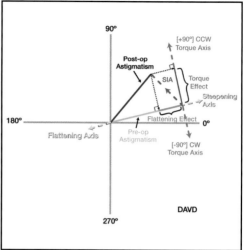

Figure 8-5. Surgical vector (polar) diagram includes the principal meridia of flattening, steepening, and torque in relation to the preoperative astigmatism meridian (selected as reference axis).

Figure 8-6. By dropping a line from the end of the SIA perpendicular to the line of the TIA, one can calculate the value of the effective SIA, or how much reduction of astigmatism (flattening) was achieved at the preoperative astigmatism axis. This value is used together with the TIA to calculate the flattening index.

ASTIGMATISM PRESENTS A COMPLEX ANALYTICAL CHALLENGE

The Alpins Method can be used for both incisional and ablative refractive procedures, with calculations performed using the ASSORT (Alpins Statistical System for Ophthalmic Refractive surgery Techniques) program, which I developed.

Any treatment that induces change in the shape of the cornea—for example, the SIA—can be resolved into 2 components: the effective proportion of the SIA that has some flattening (or steepening) effect at the axis of intended astigmatism treatment; and one I call torque, which lies at 45° clockwise or counterclockwise to the existing astigmatism and quantifies the wasted effect, or the relative ineffectiveness, of the SIA in reducing corneal astigmatism at the intended axis and results in rotation of the preoperative astigmatism. It is the effective portion of the SIA (that is, the flattening effect [FE]) that needs to be considered in any planning of future procedures. Clinically, this can be measured postoperatively by rotating the manual keratometer to the meridian of the intended astigmatic treatment and reading the magnitude of astigmatism. The difference between the preoperative astigmatism at this meridian, and the postoperative astigmatism again at this meridian, is the FE in diopters.

GRAPHICAL REPRESENTATION OF A SAMPLE CASE

Figures 8-5 and 8-6 illustrate flattening, steepening, and torque as surgical (polar) vectors and in a DAVD, respectively. In the case shown, the preoperative astigmatism

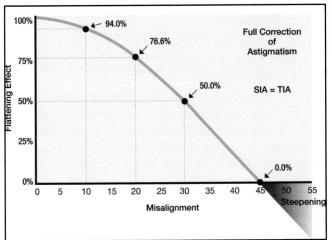

Figure 8-7. The graph shows the loss of FE of increasingly misaligned astigmatism treatment calculated by vector analysis.

was chosen as the axis under examination and all analyses performed relative to this axis. At this reference axis, which is the same for any one treatment whether performed by incisional or ablation surgery, the same astigmatic effect occurs when the greatest treatment activity to produce it (the TIA) lies at a right angle to the orientation of the existing astigmatism.

Relating back to the golf analogy, the DAVD in Figure 8-6 shows how effective the first putt (SIA) was in traveling the correct distance and direction to the cup (TIA). By dropping a line from the end of the first putt perpendicular to the line of its intended path, one can calculate the value of the effective SIA, or how much reduction of astigmatism (flattening) was achieved at the preoperative astigmatism axis. When this value is related to the TIA, a third index, called the flattening index (FI), can be calculated. The other two indices that can be calculated here are the correction index (CI) and the index of success (IOS), further described in Chapter 7.

In general terms, these three indices—CI, IOS, and FI—together with the three separate vectors—the TIA, SIA, and DV—provide a comprehensive understanding of astigmatic change and the proportion of the astigmatism treatment that has been effectively applied. The CI captures the overall astigmatism correction achieved by the SIA; the IOS is a measure of relative success derived from the DV; and the FI is calculated from the flattening effect achieved by the effective proportion of the SIA at the intended surgical meridian.

DEBATE OVER MISALIGNED TREATMENT EFFECT

There have been debates in the field related to reduction in astigmatic effect resulting from rotation or misalignment of toric IOLs (Figure 8-7). The graph is derived from vector analysis, which shows that the FE becomes smaller as a function of increasingly misaligned treatment. All other things being equal, both the SIA and CI are unaffected.

The figure shows that, when the misalignment reaches 45°, the flattening effect at the intended meridian becomes zero; that is, no measurable change in astigmatism has occurred at the treatment meridian and all the SIA effect has gone into rotating the

Sidebar 8-1

A Place for Journalistic Publications in Our Specialty

Historically, there has been a certain friction between "the journals"—that is, indexed, peer-reviewed publications—and the more journalistic types of publication, which are often written by medical reporters or even ophthalmologists, and perhaps reviewed by a medical or nonphysician editor prior to publication.[20] This clash was probably more acrimonious during the late 1970s and 1980s when such journalistic publications first appeared. Today, these different types of publications seem to have found a level of peaceful coexistence, although economic competition will forever be a factor in the operation of publications. Interestingly, technology has moved the two ends of the spectrum—thoughtful peer-reviewed scientific publishing and "medical newspapers"—closer together, as all viable publishing operations have adopted social media, blogs, "rapid publication," email alerts, etc, enabled by the Internet. We've also noted that many individuals considered leaders in our field now serve simultaneously on the editorial boards, review boards, section review boards, and other such panels associated with both types of publications.

I bring it up to acknowledge a certain fact not always discussed publically—or comfortably—among those who publish. Certainly, I have been helped greatly by editors and reviewers of our great and grand peer-reviewed publications—leaders such as Doug Koch, of the *Journal of Cataract & Refractive Surgery,* and Emanuel Rosen, a founder of the European Society of Cataract and Refractive Surgeons (ESCRS) and longtime editor of ESCRS publications. There are others too numerous to mention (and others who will be mentioned elsewhere), and reviewers who literally have helped me shape the Alpins Method into what it is. But I've also been helped by people involved with the "non–peer-reviewed" publications as an interviewee or author of countless "news" articles and an eager participant in scores of meetings and roundtables. I unabashedly enjoyed the camaraderie I found there with my peers, who likewise participated.

Some staff members of the medical newspapers, such as Keith Croes, former editor-in-chief of *Ocular Surgery News*, appeared to intuitively understand from the outset how the Alpins Method would one day become a standard in astigmatism analysis and reporting, as it has become in the *Journal of Cataract & Refractive Surgery,*[13] the *Journal of Refractive Surgery,*[14-16] and *Ophthalmology*.[12] Keith and others at *Ocular Surgery News*, *Ophthalmology Times*, and many other non–peer-reviewed publications through the years, have provided encouragement, feedback, and support. I value their role as a platform for informal discussion and a valuable tool to get a quick look at new developments in the field, and I thank them all. Rochelle Nataloni, Tim Donald, Maxine Lipner, David Mullin, Bruce Wallace, MD, Lynda Charters, Brad Fundingsland, Sean Hanahan, Paula Moyer, Leslie Sabbagh, and others were among them.

preoperative astigmatism. Beyond 45°, the FE becomes negative and astigmatism has increased (steepening). However, that amount of decrease in flattening effect brought on by misalignment does not conform to a near-linear relationship suggested by other authors. Vector analysis shows that, at 15° off axis, 13.6% of the flattening effect is lost.[4] Others have suggested that up to 50% of effect is lost at 15° off axis.[17-19] I believe this to be a significant overstatement of the loss of flattening effect caused by misalignment and this can be noted clinically where a misalignment of a toric IOL is more forgiving. Vector analysis indicates that treatment would need to be 30° off axis to yield a 50% loss of effect.[4]

WHEN REFRACTIVE AND CORNEAL ASTIGMATISM DISAGREE

The Alpins Method provides an analytical approach that can be applied independently to astigmatism measured topographically, keratometrically, or by manifest, cycloplegic, and wavefront refraction. As with the description in Chapter 5, where axis differences exist between the two modes of measurement—corneal or refractive—an on-axis correction based on one will cause an off-axis correction of the other—the non-zero target—which should be kept in mind. My method of determining an "optimal approach" can also be used, where the treatment axis does not coincide with either the refractive or topographic meridians, but still leaves the eye with the least possible astigmatism in the most favorable orientation.[2,3,8]

In addition to the optimal approach, vector analysis of flattening, steepening, and torque is useful in other situations where the intended treatment axis does not coincide with the preoperative meridian of astigmatism. This occurs in cataract surgery when a temporal incision is performed, but the steepest corneal meridian is oriented elsewhere. A discrepancy between refractive and corneal astigmatism magnitudes and/or axes is also relatively common in patients receiving excimer laser astigmatic treatment.

Flattening, steepening, and torque are useful in other situations, such as determining:

- The functional effect of incisional or ablative procedures; that is, when a treatment placed at one meridian acts functionally as though it were at a different meridian.
- A treatment's steepening/flattening effect at any axis of interest.
- A treatment's flattening effect at the preoperative steep meridian.
- The net astigmatism change at the polar axes (with-the-rule and against-the-rule); this is done by using 90° as the reference axis.

The reader is referred to my 1997 publication,[4] which describes these applications in great detail. The title of my 1997 publication uses the terms flattening, steepening, and torque, and describes them in detail as well.[4] Although they are sometimes used interchangeably, in my mind, there is a clear distinction between rotation and torque (Sidebar 8-2).

Sidebar 8-2
Letting Go of the Merry-Go-Round

In my mind, there is a distinction between rotation and torque. For example, after an astigmatic treatment is applied to the cornea, there may still be astigmatism that has rotated to a different axis and has a different magnitude. If this resulting astigmatism needs to be rotated, a clockwise or counterclockwise torque force must be applied, as appropriate.

One analogy I've used to illustrate this distinction is that of a spinning merry-go-round. The spin is rotation, with the passengers keeping a consistent distance from the rotating center. If passengers let go, they will spin off at a tangent to the circumference, 90° to the radius of the merry-go-round, in the direction of torque, not rotation, when the grip is lost. Passengers are forced to hang on by the tangential (45×2=90) force in the direction of torque, increasing their distance from the center.

CLINICAL APPLICATIONS

Using the methodology I have described, favorable changes at the preoperative astigmatism meridian are quantified by FE and ineffective changes are evaluated by torque. Clinically, incisions used in cataract surgery or limbal relaxing incisions should be analyzed using flattening, steepening, and torque parameters. Postoperative corneal astigmatism and correction index should be measured for each case to consequently adjust technique if required. The astigmatic effect of any group of incisions at one particular meridian is best quantified by their mean FE to determine their average astigmatic activity for toric implant calculation.[21] The SIA is the total change that is likely occurring at a meridian away from the incision and would overestimate this parameter of effective change.

I believe my approach to flattening, steepening, and torque significantly contributes to our understanding of induced astigmatic change and enables integrated analysis of all changes applicable to keratometry, topography, or refraction values.

REFERENCES

1. Alpins N, Stamatelatos G. Chapter 24: The Cornea - Part X: Treatment and analysis of astigmatism during the laser era. In: Boyd BF, ed. *Modern Ophthalmology: The Highlights.* New Delhi, India: J.P. Medical Ltd; 2010:381-404.

2. Alpins NA. A new method of analyzing vectors for changes in astigmatism. *J Cataract Refract Surg.* 1993;19(4):524-533.

3. Alpins NA. New method of targeting vectors to treat astigmatism. *J Cataract Refract Surg.* 1997;23(1):65-75.

4. Alpins NA. Vector analysis of astigmatism changes by flattening, steepening, and torque. *J Cataract Refract Surg.* 1997;23(10):1503-1514.

5. MC, Alpins N, Verma S, Stamatelatos G, Arbelaez JG, Arba-Mosquera S. Clinical outcomes of LASIK with an aberration-neutral profile centred on the corneal vertex comparing vector planning to manifest refraction planning for the treatment of myopic astigmatism. *J Cataract Refract Surg*. In press.

6. Alpins NA. Topographic disparity: a useful new measure of irregular astigmatism. *Ocular Surgery News*. July 15, 1999:8.

7. Alpins NA. Flattening, steepening, and torque are crucial points in astigmatism surgery. *Ocular Surgery News*. June 1, 1999:19.

8. Alpins NA. Corneal versus refractive astigmatism: integrated analysis. *Ocular Surgery News*. June 15, 1999:44.

9. Alpins NA. The treatment of irregular astigmatism. *Ocular Surgery News*. July 1, 1999:6.

10. Alpins NA. Vector analysis of astigmatism correction: the Alpins method. *Ocular Surgery News*. May 15, 1999:14.

11. Naeser K. Surgically induced astigmatism: distinguishing between dioptric vectors and non-vectors [letter]. *J Refract Surg*. 2015;31(5):349-350.

12. Author Information Pack. American Academy of Ophthalmology Web site. https://www.elsevier.com/wps/find/journaldescription.cws_home/620418?generatepdf=true. Accessed January 19, 2016.

13. Information for Authors. American Society of Cataract and Refractive Surgery Web site http://www.jcrsjournal.org/content/authorinfo#info. Accessed September 1, 2016.

14. Reinstein DZ, Archer TJ, Randleman JB. JRS standard for reporting astigmatism outcomes of refractive surgery [editorial]. *J Refract Surg*. 2014;30(10):654-659.

15. Reinstein DZ, Randleman JB, Archer TJ. JRS standard for reporting outcomes of intraocular lens based refractive surgery. *J Refract Surg*. 2017;22(4):218-222.

16. Reinstein DZ, Archer TJ, Srinivasan S, Mamalis N, Kohnen T, Dupps Jr WJ, Randleman JB. Standard for reporting refractive outcomes of intraocular lens-based refractive surgery. *J Cataract Refract Surg*. 2017;43(4); 435-439.

17. Hirnschall N, Maedel S, Weber M, Findl O. Rotational stability of a single-piece toric acrylic intraocular lens: a pilot study. *Am J Ophthalmol*. 2014;157(2):405-411.

18. Mencucci R, Favuzza E, Guerra F, Giacomelli G, Menchini U. Clinical outcomes and rotational stability of a 4-haptic toric intraocular lens in myopic eyes. *J Cataract Refract Surg*. 2014;40(9):1479-1487.

19. Novis C. Astigmatism and toric intraocular lenses. *Curr Opin Ophthalmol*. 2000;11(1):47-50.

20. Croes KJ. Ophthalmologists in the 'news' [letter]. *Arch Ophthalmol*. 1995;113(8):968-969.

21. Alpins N, Ong JKY, Stamatelatos G. Asymmetric corneal flattening effect after small incision cataract surgery. *J Refract Surg*. 2016;32(9):598-603.

Chapter 9

Ocular Residual Astigmatism
When Zero Is Not the Target

REFRACTIVE AND CORNEAL ASTIGMATISM: DISAGREEABLE

Only rarely are refractive and corneal astigmatism values in complete agreement with one another.[1-8] They usually disagree both in axis and magnitude. When this difference is large, it might catch the practitioner's attention, perhaps initiating the question of what, if anything, should be done about it.

Duke-Elder called this difference residual astigmatism. He noted that the greatest contributor to the total astigmatism of the eye, as measured by refraction, was the anterior surface of the cornea. The residual astigmatism, he wrote, was caused by the posterior surface of the cornea and the anterior and posterior surfaces of the crystalline lens, as well as any decentration or variability of the refractive index of the lens.[1]

Although the magnitude of residual astigmatism in most patients is small, Duke-Elder cautioned that residual astigmatism "by no means [should be] neglected." He cited other work that showed average corneal astigmatism of 1.04 D in a large series of young adults, and an average residual astigmatism of 0.61 D, ranging up to 8 D of corneal astigmatism and 4.25 D of residual astigmatism. He noted "[t]he significant degree of residual astigmatism is sufficient commentary on the inefficiency of the clinical correction of astigmatic errors estimated by keratometry alone."[1]

I described the residual astigmatism vectorially, with magnitude and axis orientation—more specifically, the vectorial difference between corneal and refractive astigmatism calculated at the corneal plane—and so introduced the term ocular residual astigmatism[2,9,10] (ORA) to differentiate ORA from residual astigmatism as commonly used to mean the astigmatism remaining after surgery.[9-16] The astigmatism should be better termed "surgical residual astigmatism" or SRA. In addition to the eye's optical properties from the posterior cornea through the crystalline lens as described by Duke-Elder, I believe that at least some proportion of ORA must arise from retinal tilt and perception as experienced in the visual cortex—the so-called eye-brain interface.[6,8,9,12,13,17] Confusion about the definition of ORA and other vector calculations has been common in the field,[7,11,18-26] although some consensus appears to be emerging[27-30,31] (Sidebar 9-1).

Alpins N. *Practical Astigmatism:*
Planning and Analysis (pp 65-76).
© 2018 SLACK Incorporated.

Sidebar 9-1

Ocular Residual Astigmatism
Adopting Standard Terminology

The term residual astigmatism was coined and defined by Duke-Elder in 1970.[1] I described the parameter vectorially, with magnitude and axis orientation, and introduced the term ORA[9] to differentiate it from residual astigmatism, which has been commonly used to mean the astigmatism remaining after surgery.[11]

Several terms have been used, inappropriately, as a substitute for ORA; they include intraocular, lenticular, noncorneal, and internal astigmatism. Although these ocular phenomena undoubtedly are involved in the calculation of ORA, I use every opportunity to recommend they be avoided, as the ORA also has nonoptical perceptual components that contribute to measured cylinder.[2,9-11] Some people also use the abbreviation ORA informally when referring to a number of available ophthalmic biometric and/or medical devices developed and named after the scientific publication of ORA in 1997.[9] This is another potential source of confusion that should be avoided; that is, the full names of these devices should be used as opposed to simply calling them "the ORA."

A non–peer-reviewed article[32] in the *Journal of Refractive Surgery (JRS)*, apparently submitted by a committee of the American National Standards Institute (ANSI), muddied the water for many investigators by renaming and publishing indices I had developed previously[2,10,33] (Table 9-1). The ANSI paper spurred a flurry of letters to the editor.[18-20,22]

Even after the corrective letters to the editor, the discredited ANSI terminology continued to appear in the literature. Even as recently as 2016, St. Clair and colleagues[26] used the erroneous ANSI nomenclature. In some cases, as with Trivizki et al,[25] I was able to correct the record[24]; however, I'm sure there are other papers extant in the literature that perpetrate the ANSI debacle.

Obviously, confusing terminology related to ORA and other vector calculations has been widespread in the field.[7,11,18-22,24-26,32] Fortunately, the major cataract and refractive surgical journals[27-30,31] have adopted the many terms and graphical representations described by the Alpins Method as standard, so we expect future articles that report astigmatism results to be more accurate, consistent, and accessible to researchers. I offer special thanks to the editors *JRS*, who in 2014, made it the first ophthalmic journal to adopt Alpins Method terminology and graphical representations as the standard for future reporting.[29] I am fairly confident now that astigmatism terminology will settle down to its standard format as we go about the art and science of improving our patients' vision.

Table 9-1	
Alpins Method	**ANSI**
Target induced astigmatism vector (TIA)	Intended refractive correction (IRC)
Surgically induced astigmatism vector (SIA)	Surgically induced refractive correction (SIRC)
Magnitude of error	Error of magnitude
Angle of error	Error of angle
Difference vector (DV)	Error vector
Correction index	Correction ratio
Index of success	Error ratio

Abbreviation: ANSI, American National Standards Institute.

JRS recommended use of the Alpins Method terminology,[2,10,33] which was published prior to identical concepts with modified names, developed by a committee of the American National Standards Institute.[34] Reprinted with permission from Reinstein DZ, Archer TJ, Randleman JB. JRS standard for reporting astigmatism outcomes of refractive surgery [editorial]. *J Refract Surg.* 2014;30(10):654-659.

ORA may be abnormally high in some pathological conditions, such as keratoconus[3,32,33,35] or ectasia after laser-assisted in situ keratomileusis (LASIK).[36] ORA also has the potential to contribute to diagnoses of some corneal disorders.[37]

Figures 9-1 and 9-2 are conceptual models of low and high ORA, respectively, before and after LASIK. One group used these ray-tracing principles in an attempt to explain the clinical differences they observed in patients with low and high preoperative ORA.[6] The figures are not an actual representation of any specific case, and assume that the ORA is lenticular only.

In the normal population, the majority of eyes have an ORA between 0 and 1 D, ranging up to 2 D.[2-9,37-40] Recent studies have found ORA ranging from 0.73 D to 1.06 D prior to LASIK (Table 9-2).

In the years ahead, the continued advance of technology will enable more and more practitioners to better understand the role of posterior corneal astigmatism. It is known that a correlation exists between the toricity of anterior and posterior corneal surfaces in the healthy human eye, with a ratio of posterior to anterior astigmatism between 0.3 and 0.4.[41-43] The compensatory effects of the posterior corneal surface of the normal healthy eye—about 22% of the magnitude of the anterior corneal astigmatism in one study[44]—as well as the significance of the relative orientation of posterior and anterior corneal astigmatism, remain to be completely worked out. Our efforts in describing and utilizing measures we call corneal topographic astigmatism (CorT)[45] and CorT total,[46] which incorporates posterior corneal astigmatism, are described in Chapter 12. Our concept of the Vector Planning approach, described in Chapter 13, will be especially useful in patients having higher degrees of ORA.[3,4,40,47]

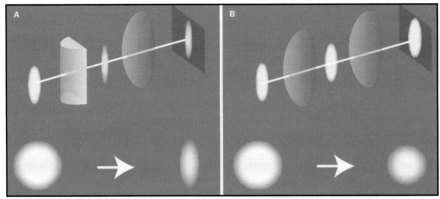

Figure 9-1. Model of an eye with low ocular residual astigmatism. (A) Preoperatively, the astigmatism is mainly on the cornea. The cornea is a cylinder, the lens is a perfect sphere, and the retinal image is a cylinder corresponding to the corneal cylinder. (B) Postoperatively, the cornea is a sphere, the lens is a sphere, and the retinal image is a perfect sphere. (Reprinted from *Journal of Cataract & Refractive Surgery*, 36/10, Kugler L, Cohen I, Haddad W, Wang MX, Efficacy of laser in situ keratomileusis in correcting anterior and non-anterior corneal astigmatism: comparative study, 8, Copyright 2010, with permission from Elsevier.)

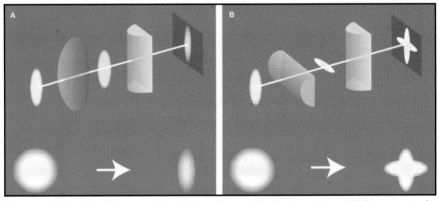

Figure 9-2. Model of an eye with high ocular residual astigmatism. (A) Preoperatively, the astigmatism is mainly lenticular. The cornea is a sphere, the lens is a cylinder, and the retinal image is a cylinder corresponding to the lenticular cylinder. (B) Postoperatively, the cornea is a cylinder, the lens is a cylinder, and the retinal image is blurred and distorted. (Reprinted from *Journal of Cataract & Refractive Surgery*, 36/10, Kugler L, Cohen I, Haddad W, Wang MX, Efficacy of laser in situ keratomileusis in correcting anterior and non-anterior corneal astigmatism: comparative study, 8, Copyright 2010, with permission from Elsevier.)

IF THERE'S AN OCULAR RESIDUAL ASTIGMATISM, THERE'S A NONZERO TARGET

The difference between refractive and corneal astigmatism can be seen on double-angle vector diagrams (DAVDs), which depict ORA and the nonzero target (Figure 9-3). As described above, ORA is defined as the vectorial difference between corneal and refractive astigmatism calculated at the corneal plane.[2,9,10]

As with most, the patient in Figure 9-3 has a difference between corneal and refractive astigmatism and thus, by definition, has ORA. The DAVDs illustrate the situation

Table 9-2

Studies Reporting ORA Calculated Prior to LASIK

Study	N	Magnitude (mean, D)	Range (D)	Levels of Magnitude
Frings A et al[5]	2991	0.75 ± 0.39	0.00 to 2.00	1372 (46%) with ORA of 1.00 D or more
Qian YS et al[7]	192	0.79 ± 0.36*	–	91 patients with high ORA
Alpins N and Stamatelatos G[4]	21 eyes in 14 patients	1.00 ± 0.16 (WF) 1.06 ± 0.23 (WF&VP)	0.80 to 1.32 (WF) 0.77 to 1.18 (WF&VP)	–
Alpins N and Stamatelatos G[3]	45 eyes with forme fruste or mild keratoconus	1.34 ± 1.00	0.23 to 4.37	–
Alpins N[10]	Dataset of 100	0.73 ± 0.43	0.72 to 0.74	–
Alpins NA[9]	Dataset of 100	0.81 ± 0.05†	0.01 to 2.32	34 (34%) with ORA of > 1.00 D

*Called lenticular astigmatism in this study.
†Standard error of the mean.
Abbreviations: D, diopters; LASIK, laser-assisted in situ keratomileusis; WF, wavefront aberrometry; WF&VP, wavefront aberrometry plus Vector Planning approach.

where astigmatism treatment is targeted 100% by topography (A), 100% by refraction (B), or at some intermediate point between topography and refraction using the Vector Planning approach (C). Note, that when astigmatism treatment is targeted solely on topography (A), there is—simultaneously and inescapably—a target refraction that is not zero. Similarly, if one targets treatment 100% on refraction, as shown in diagram B, there is a simultaneous and inescapable target topography that is not zero. This is the nonzero target.

The concept I call optimal treatment is based on the surgical emphasis graph and typical ORA calculation provided as an example in Figure 9-4A and 9-4B, respectively.[9] As ORA is the absolute, inescapable, minimal amount of astigmatism that can remain in the eye after LASIK, the target induced astigmatism vector (TIA), when maximal and optimal, terminates on the ORA line. The surgeon can choose a TIA that puts 100% emphasis on refraction, 100% on topography, or a combination emphasis at any intermediate point on the ORA.

Figure 9-3. (A) DAVDs demonstrate, the treatment needed to achieve a spherical cornea by topographic (T) values; (B), the treatment needed to achieve a spherical refraction (R); and (C), a combination treatment that nonetheless lies on the ORA vector of minimal achievable astigmatism. To achieve minimal astigmatism with maximal correction, the TIA must terminate on the ORA line.[9]

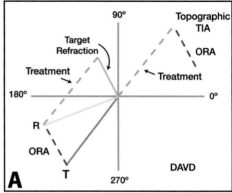

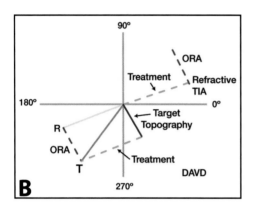

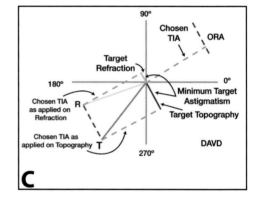

Figure 9-4A is a linear relationship meant only to suggest laser settings that put a greater emphasis on refractive astigmatism the closer the remaining/targeted corneal astigmatism is to 90° (with-the-rule). If the meridian of target topography is 90°, 100% of the treatment emphasis will be devoted to the correction of refractive astigmatism. If the meridian of target topography is 180°, 100% of the treatment emphasis will be devoted to correcting the topographic astigmatism to achieve a spherical cornea. Optimal treatment seeks to achieve less corneal astigmatism than if treating by refraction alone, with an attempt to influence its orientation favorably[33,48,49] by minimizing potentially unfavorable results.

The Alpins Method, developed in many peer-reviewed articles over the years,[2,4,9,12,51,52] is programmed into a commercially available ophthalmic surgical analysis system called ASSORT[53] (Alpins Statistical System for Ophthalmic Refractive surgery Techniques). The ASSORT program calculates ORA and helps plan and analyze the results of refractive, corneal, and cataract surgical procedures.[3,4,40,54-60] ORA can also be calculated using iASSORT, a scaled-down version of the ASSORT program that interfaces with most of the leading tomographers and topographers (CSO Sirius, Oculus Pentacam, Ziemer Galilei, Zeiss Atlas, Nidek OPD III, and others). The ASSORT programs, and various free online calculators, are described further in Chapter 24.

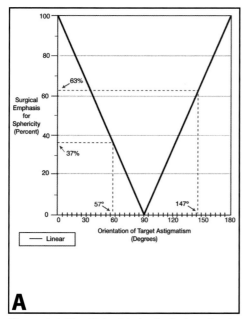
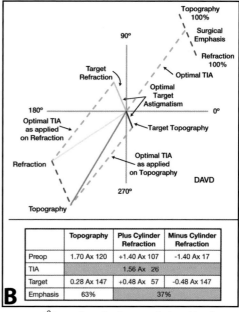

	Topography	Plus Cylinder Refraction	Minus Cylinder Refraction
Preop	1.70 Ax 120	+1.40 Ax 107	-1.40 Ax 17
TIA		1.56 Ax 26	
Target	0.28 Ax 147	+0.48 Ax 57	-0.48 Ax 147
Emphasis	63%	37%	

Figure 9-4. The Alpins Method calculates "optimal treatment"[9] based on the linear relationship shown in graph A. Future research may determine that the actual relationship is nonlinear or otherwise varies from the graph shown. In this example, the meridian of target topography is 147°, which lies 57° from a with-the-rule orientation of 90°. Using this linear relationship, the surgeon may decide to apportion 57° of 90° (63.3%) emphasis to a topography-based goal of zero astigmatism (147° intersects the linear emphasis line at 63%). This results in a 37% emphasis on the correction of refractive astigmatism. Graph B is a DAVD of the optimal TIA and treatment parameters.

OCULAR RESIDUAL ASTIGMATISM AND VISUAL OUTCOMES

For patients with high ORA (> 1.00 D), a practitioner should consider finding an answer to the question posed above: What, if anything, should be done about it?

The efficacy of refractive laser treatment is better in eyes with low ORA compared with high ORA.[3,4,6-8,17,40,54,61,62] Additionally, the magnitude of ORA has been related to the quality of postoperative vision.[63-66]

Two groups—Kugler et al[6] and Qian et al[7]—approached the question in different ways, providing an interesting contrast. In a retrospective case series, Kugler et al[6] found that LASIK was twice as efficacious in correcting refractive astigmatism in a low-ORA group (ORA/refractive astigmatism > 1.0) than in a high-ORA group (ORA/refractive astigmatism > 1.0).[6] In a retrospective study, Qian et al[7] found that LASIK was less effective in correcting refractive astigmatism when the astigmatism was located mainly in the internal optics.[7] In both of these papers, the authors recommended that topography and refractive astigmatism values should be considered together in surgical planning for patients with high preoperative ORA. This approach, which we call the Vector Planning technique, is further described in Chapter 13.

Kugler et al[17] also analyzed ORA by age (Figure 9-5). The authors speculate that the significantly higher ORA values in patients older than 45 years may be due to age-related changes in the crystalline lens as dysfunctional lens syndrome progresses. The findings suggest that, in older patients with high ORA, an intraocular or lens-based

Figure 9-5. Ocular residual astigmatism increases with age ($P \leq .0001$).[17] (Reprinted with permission from Kugler L, Crews J, Morgan L. Ocular Residual Astigmatism. *CRST.* 2014;14(8):16-18.)

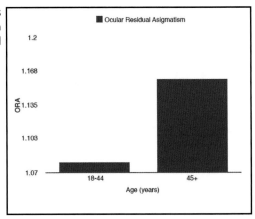

refractive procedure may be preferred over a corneal procedure. Laser treatment of the cornea in these patients may lead to the ORA being permanently imprinted on the cornea (at a meridian 90° away from the calculated ORA axis to neutralize it on the cornea). Furthermore, they note, as the crystalline lens continues to change with age, a higher enhancement rate can be expected in these patients.

Reinstein et al[8] conducted a retrospective analysis that categorized patients into a variety of low-, medium-, and high-ORA groups, using ratios (ORA/manifest refractive cylinder [MRC]) and ORA magnitude, matched and unmatched for MRC, with some groups subdivided for magnitude of corneal astigmatism (CA). (Note—The studies by Kugler et al[6] and Qian et al[7] did not match for refractive cylinder. The Qian study also included eyes with 0.25 D of astigmatism treatment. Both these factors introduce some bias to the results.) The study by Reinstein et al[8] found that the accuracy of refractive astigmatism correction was worse in eyes with high ORA. The worst results were found in eyes with high ORA and high CA. This may be related to the fact that astigmatic ablation profiles and simulated keratometry values assume astigmatism to be orthogonal.

The high ORA in this study was due to low refractive cylinder and high corneal astigmatism. The treatments were based on refractive parameters alone and were thus small, so patients were left with excessive corneal astigmatism as a result. Although corneal astigmatism is orthogonal in most eyes, a certain percentage may have asymmetric and nonorthogonal corneal astigmatism, where superior and inferior hemidivisions have different axes. In these cases, corneal astigmatism calculated using simulated keratometry would not accurately represent the corneal astigmatism. Simulated keratometry is also more likely to be misaligned with the MRC, producing a higher calculated ORA.

A parameter we have described, called topographic disparity (TD),[10,67,68] detailed in Chapter 16, is more helpful and accurate than simulated keratometry for asymmetric corneal astigmatism. We have shown CorT, derived from astigmatism vectors for each Placido ring on topography, also corresponds better to MRC than simulated keratometry and other common measures.[45] The Vector Planning approach in these cases—taking into account ORA, MRC, corneal astigmatism, and TIA—will help minimize the resultant anterior corneal astigmatism[7,9,40] while also effectively reducing refractive cylinder.

THE FUTURE OF OCULAR RESIDUAL ASTIGMATISM

ORA appears to be enjoying a growing, fundamental acceptance in the ophthalmic peer-reviewed literature. The basic differences in the tools we use to measure corneal and refractive astigmatism may never be reconciled—the former based on an ever-more-accurate reconstruction of corneal shape made possible by topography and keratometry; the latter resulting from the subjective experience of the entire visual system, from the front corneal surface back to the visual cortex of the brain, and the many interfaces in between, or indeed from wavefront aberrometry or just the eye itself. ORA as a significant phenomenon, affecting the outcome of astigmatic refractive surgery, can only persist. The use of a Vector Planning approach as a systematic method linking corneal and refractive astigmatism, calculating prior to surgery the minimum amount of astigmatism that can be achieved for the eye, is destined to become routine for preoperative assessment and optimization of treatment.

The steady expansion of ORA in the literature, and its importance in optimizing final visual results, seems to have made inroads in dampening the knee-jerk question: Why not use refraction as the only treatment parameter for both cylinder and sphere? The answer now is simple: The data do not support it. Applying astigmatism treatment exclusively on the refractive cylinder magnitude and axis can leave an excessive amount of corneal astigmatism,[10] leading to increased aberrations and a reduction in the quality of vision achieved.[4] In my experience, about 7% of patients have an ORA that could result in increased corneal astigmatism after LASIK if the target is based solely on refraction.[9]

DON'T MAKE A SPECTACLE OF THE CORNEA

The cornea is not a spectacle lens but human tissue. The potential exists for increased spherical aberrations with degradation of the perceived image.[69] The eye's optical system, independent of spectacle correction, will continue to be significantly influenced by the optimal regularity and shape of the anterior corneal surface. What is often overlooked by surgeons is that glasses may no longer be necessary after refractive surgery if the spherical equivalent being targeted is zero; however, the patient must "wear" their cornea for the rest of their lives.

One meta-analysis found that the overall patient satisfaction rate after primary LASIK surgery was 95.4% (2097 of 2198 subjects); the range of patient satisfaction for the 19 articles in the meta-analysis was 87.2% to 100%. The patient satisfaction rate after myopic LASIK was 95.3% (1811 of 1901 patients).[68] Disgruntled LASIK patients, who might inhabit the 5% or so of unsatisfied patients, have little trouble finding reinforcement for their negative views on the Internet[32] and are widely invited to contact the Food and Drug Administration with reports of adverse events. Ignoring the nonzero target for corneal astigmatism, an unavoidable byproduct of treating only the refractive error, may account for many unhappy LASIK patients with or without 20/20 visual acuity.

In my opinion, it is likely that unrecognized high preoperative ORA often accompanies unhappy LASIK patients. People with high preoperative ORA can be better managed if their expectations are lowered as to their postoperative results and/or they are treated with a Vector Planning approach, which optimizes possible postoperative results, reducing total remaining corneal and refractive astigmatism.

REFERENCES

1. Duke-Elder SS. *System of Ophthalmology - Ophthalmic Optics and Refraction*. St Louis, MO: Mosby; 1970.

2. Alpins NA. A new method of analyzing vectors for changes in astigmatism. *J Cataract Refract Surg*. 1993;19(4):524-533.

3. Alpins N, Stamatelatos G. Customized photoastigmatic refractive keratectomy using combined topographic and refractive data for myopia and astigmatism in eyes with forme fruste and mild keratoconus. *J Cataract Refract Surg*. 2007;33(4):591-602.

4. Alpins N, Stamatelatos G. Clinical outcomes of laser in situ keratomileusis using combined topography and refractive wavefront treatments for myopic astigmatism. *J Cataract Refract Surg*. 2008;34(8):1250-1259.

5. Frings A, Katz T, Steinberg J, Druchkiv V, Richard G, Linke SJ. Ocular residual astigmatism: effects of demographic and ocular parameters in myopic laser in situ keratomileusis. *J Cataract Refract Surg*. 2014;40(2):232-238.

6. Kugler L, Cohen I, Haddad W, Wang MX. Efficacy of laser in situ keratomileusis in correcting anterior and non-anterior corneal astigmatism: comparative study. *J Cataract Refract Surg*. 2010;36(10):1745-1752.

7. Qian YS, Huang J, Liu R, et al. Influence of internal optical astigmatism on the correction of myopic astigmatism by LASIK. *J Refract Surg*. 2011;27(12):863-868.

8. Reinstein DZ, Archer TJ, Piñero DP, Gobbe M, Carp GI. Comparison of the predictability of refractive cylinder by laser in situ keratomileusis in eyes with low and high ocular residual astigmatism. *J Cataract Refract Surg*. 2015;41(7):1383-1392.

9. Alpins NA. New method of targeting vectors to treat astigmatism. *J Cataract Refract Surg*. 1997;23(1):65-75.

10. Alpins N. Astigmatism analysis by the Alpins method. *J Cataract Refract Surg*. 2001;27(1):31-49.

11. Alio JL, Alpins N. Excimer laser correction of astigmatism: consistent terminology for better outcomes. *J Refract Surg*. 2014;30(5):294-295.

12. Alpins N, Stamatelatos G. Chapter 24: The Cornea - Part X: Treatment and analysis of astigmatism during the laser era. In: Boyd BF, ed. *Modern Ophthalmology: The Highlights*. New Delhi, India: J.P. Medical Ltd; 2010:381-404.

13. Alpins NA. Wavefront technology: a new advance that fails to answer old questions on corneal vs. refractive astigmatism correction. *J Refract Surg*. 2002;18(6):737-739.

14. Alpins NA, Stamatelatos G. Combined wavefront and topography approach to refractive surgery treatments. In: Wang M, editor. *Corneal Topography in the Wavefront Era: A Guide for Clinical Application*. Thorofare, NJ: SLACK Incorporated; 2006:139-143.

15. Kohnen T. Combining wavefront and topography data for excimer laser surgery: the future of customized ablation? *J Cataract Refract Surg*. 2004;30(2):285-286.

16. Tejedor J, Guirao A. Agreement between refractive and corneal astigmatism in pseudophakic eyes. *Cornea*. 2013;32(6):783-790.

17. Kugler L, Crews J, Morgan L. *Ocular residual astigmatism. Cataract and Refractive Surgery Today*. 2014;16-8.

18. Alpins N. Terms used for the analysis of astigmatism [letter]. *J Refract Surg*. 2006;22(6):528-529.

19. Goggin M. More on astigmatism analysis [letter]. *J Refract Surg*. 2007;23(5):430-431.

20. Masket S. Special articles and peer review [letter]. *J Refract Surg*. 2007;23(2):115.

21. Pena-Garcia P, Alio JL, Vega-Estrada A, Barraquer RI. Internal, corneal, and refractive astigmatism as prognostic factors for intrastromal corneal ring segment implantation in mild to moderate keratoconus. *J Cataract Refract Surg*. 2014;40:1633-1644.

22. Pinero DP. Terminology and referencing of astigmatic vector analysis [letter]. *J Cataract Refract Surg*. 2013;39(11):1792.

23. Kunert KS, Russmann C, Blum M, Sluyterman VLG. Vector analysis of myopic astigmatism corrected by femtosecond refractive lenticule extraction. *J Cataract Refract Surg*. 2013;39(5):759-769.

24. Alpins N. Astigmatism terminology and source references [letter]. *J Cataract Refract Surg.* 2016;42(4):643.

25. Trivizki O, Levinger E, Levinger S. Correction ratio and vector analysis of femtosecond laser arcuate keratotomy for the correction of post-mushroom profile keratoplasty astigmatism. *J Cataract Refract Surg.* 2015;41(9):1973-1979.

26. St Clair RM, Sharma A, Huang D, et al. Development of a nomogram for femtosecond laser astigmatic keratotomy for astigmatism after keratoplasty. *J Cataract Refract Surg.* 2016;42(4):556-562.

27. Author Information Pack. American Academy of Ophthalmology Web site. https://www.elsevier.com/wps/find/journaldescription.cws_home/620418?generatepdf=true. Accessed January 19, 2016.

28. Information for Authors. American Society of Cataract and Refractive Surgery Web site. http://www.jcrsjournal.org/content/authorinfo#info. Accessed September 1, 2016.

29. Reinstein DZ, Archer TJ, Randleman JB. JRS standard for reporting astigmatism outcomes of refractive surgery [editorial]. *J Refract Surg.* 2014;30(10):654-659.

30. Reinstein DZ, Randleman JB, Archer TJ, et al. JRS standard for reporting outcomes of intraocular lens based refractive surgery. *J Refract Surg.* 2017;33(4):218-222.

31. Reinstein DZ, Archer TJ, Srinivasan S, Mamalis N, Kohnen T, Dupps Jr WJ, Randleman JB. Standard for reporting refractive outcomes of intraocular lens-based refractive surgery. *J Cataract Refract Surg.* 2017;43(4):435-439.

32. Pinero DP, Alio JL, Tomas J, Maldonado MJ, Teus MA, Barraquer RI. Vector analysis of evolutive corneal astigmatic changes in keratoconus. *Invest Ophthalmol Vis Sci.* 2011;52(7):4054-4062.

33. Alio JL, Pinero DP, Aleson A, et al. Keratoconus-integrated characterization considering anterior corneal aberrations, internal astigmatism, and corneal biomechanics. *J Cataract Refract Surg.* 2011;37(3):552-568.

34. Eydelman MB, Drum B, Holladay J, et al. Standardized analyses of correction of astigmatism by laser systems that reshape the cornea. *J Refract Surg.* 2006;22(1):81-95.

35. Martinez-Abad A, Pinero DP, Ruiz-Fortes P, Artola A. Evaluation of the diagnostic ability of vector parameters characterizing the corneal astigmatism and regularity in clinical and subclinical keratoconus. *Cont Lens Anterior Eye.* 2017;40(2):88-96.

36. Pinero DP, Alio JL, Barraquer RI, Uceda-Montanes A, Murta J. Clinical characterization of corneal ectasia after myopic laser in situ keratomileusis based on anterior corneal aberrations and internal astigmatism. *J Cataract Refract Surg.* 2011;37(7):1291-1299.

37. Pinero DP, Ruiz-Fortes P, Perez-Cambrodi RJ, Mateo V, Artola A. Ocular residual astigmatism and topographic disparity vector indexes in normal healthy eyes. *Cont Lens Anterior Eye.* 2014;37(1):49-54.

38. Srivannaboon S. Internal astigmatism and its correlation to corneal and refractive astigmatism. *J Med Assoc Thai.* 2003;86(2):166-171.

39. Bragheeth MA, Dua HS. Effect of refractive and topographic astigmatic axis on LASIK correction of myopic astigmatism. *J Refract Surg.* 2005;21(3):269-275.

40. Arbelaez MC, Alpins N, Verma S, Stamatelatos G, Arbelaez JG, Arba-Mosquera S. Clinical outcomes of LASIK with an aberration-neutral profile centred on the corneal vertex comparing vector planning to manifest refraction planning for the treatment of myopic astigmatism. *J Cataract Refract Surg.* In press.

41. Mas D, Espinosa J, Domenech B, Perez J, Kasprzak H, Illueca C. Correlation between the dioptric power, astigmatism and surface shape of the anterior and posterior corneal surfaces. *Ophthalmic Physiol Opt.* 2009;29(3):219-226.

42. Montalban R, Pinero DP, Javaloy J, Alio JL. Correlation of the corneal toricity between anterior and posterior corneal surfaces in the normal human eye. *Cornea.* 2013;32(6):791-798.

43. Oshika T, Tomidokoro A, Tsuji H. Regular and irregular refractive powers of the front and back surfaces of the cornea. *Exp Eye Res.* 1998;67(4):443-447.

44. Atchison DA, Markwell EL, Kasthurirangan S, Pope JM, Smith G, Swann PG. Age-related changes in optical and biometric characteristics of emmetropic eyes. *J Vis.* 2008;8(4):29.

45. Alpins N, Ong JK, Stamatelatos G. New method of quantifying corneal topographic astigmatism that corresponds with manifest refractive cylinder. *J Cataract Refract Surg.* 2012;38(11):1978-1988.

46. Alpins NA, Ong JKY, Stamatelatos G. Corneal topographic astigmatism (CorT) to quantify total corneal astigmatism. *J Refract Surg.* 2015;31(3):182-186.

47. Alpins N. Combining wavefront and topography data [letter]. *J Cataract Refract Surg.* 2005;31(4):646-647.

48. Eggers H. Estimation of uncorrected visual acuity in malingerers. *Arch Ophthalmol.* 1945;33:23-27.

49. Friedman B. Acceptance of weak cylinders at paradoxic axes. *Arch Ophthalmol.* 1940;23:720-726.

50. Sawusch MR, Guyton DL. Optimal astigmatism to enhance depth of focus after cataract surgery. *Ophthalmology.* 1991;98:1025-1029.

51. Alpins NA. Vector analysis of astigmatism changes by flattening, steepening, and torque. *J Cataract Refract Surg.* 1997;23(10):1503-1514.

52. Alpins NA, Goggin M. Practical astigmatism analysis for refractive outcomes in cataract and refractive surgery. *Surv Ophthalmol.* 2004;49(1):109-122.

53. ASSORT Web site. http://www.assort.com. Accessed April 22, 2014.

54. Alpins NA, Tabin GC, Adams LM, Aldred GF, Kent DG, Taylor HR. Refractive versus corneal changes after photorefractive keratectomy for astigmatism. *J Refract Surg.* 1998;14(4):386-396.

55. Fraenkel GE, Webber SK, Sutton GL, Lawless MA, Rogers CM. Toric laser in situ keratomileusis for myopic astigmatism using an ablatable mask. *J Refract Surg.* 1999;15(2):111-117.

56. Pinero DP, Alio JL, Teus MA, Barraquer RI, Michael R, Jimenez R. Modification and refinement of astigmatism in keratoconic eyes with intrastromal corneal ring segments. *J Cataract Refract Surg.* 2010;36(9):1562-1572.

57. Alio JL, Agdeppa MC, Pongo VC, El KB. Microincision cataract surgery with toric intraocular lens implantation for correcting moderate and high astigmatism: pilot study. *J Cataract Refract Surg.* 2010;36(1):44-52.

58. Galway G, Drury B, Cronin BG, Bourke RD. A comparison of induced astigmatism in 20- vs 25-gauge vitrectomy procedures. *Eye (Lond).* 2010;24(2):315-317.

59. Alio JL, Pinero DP, Tomas J, Plaza AB. Vector analysis of astigmatic changes after cataract surgery with implantation of a new toric multifocal intraocular lens. *J Cataract Refract Surg.* 2011;37(7):1217-1229.

60. Alio JL, Pinero DP, Tomas J, Aleson A. Vector analysis of astigmatic changes after cataract surgery with toric intraocular lens implantation. *J Cataract Refract Surg.* 2011;37(6):1038-1049.

61. Labiris G, Gatzioufas Z, Giarmoukakis A, Sideroudi H, Kozobolis V. Evaluation of the efficacy of the Allegretto Wave and the Wavefront-optimized ablation profile in non-anterior astigmatisms. *Acta Ophthalmol.* 2012;90(6):e442-e446.

62. Qian Y, Huang J, Chu R, Zhou X, Olszewski E. Influence of intraocular astigmatism on the correction of myopic astigmatism by laser-assisted subepithelial keratectomy. *J Cataract Refract Surg.* 2014;40(4):558-563.

63. Artal P, Guirao A, Berrio E, Williams DR. Compensation of corneal aberrations by the internal optics in the human eye. *J Vis.* 2001;1(1):1-8.

64. Atchison DA. Anterior corneal and internal contributions to peripheral aberrations of human eyes. *J Opt Soc Am A Opt Image Sci Vis.* 2004;21(3):355-359.

65. Le Grand Y, El Hage SG. *Physiological Optics.* New York, NY: Springer-Verlag; 1980.

66. Mrochen M, Jankov M, Bueeler M, Seiler T. Correlation between corneal and total wavefront aberrations in myopic eyes. *J Refract Surg.* 2003;19(2):104-112.

67. Alpins NA. Treatment of irregular astigmatism. *J Cataract Refract Surg.* 1998;24(5):634-646.

68. Alpins NA. Topographic disparity: a useful new measure of irregular astigmatism. *Ocular Surgery News.* July 15, 1999:8.

69. Seiler T, Reckmann W, Maloney RK. Effective spherical aberration of the cornea as a quantitative descriptor in corneal topography. *J Cataract Refract Surg.* 1993;19(Suppl):155-165.

70. Solomon KD, Fernandez de Castro LE, Sandoval HP et al. LASIK world literature review: quality of life and patient satisfaction. *Ophthalmology.* 2009;116(4):691-701.

71. The truth behind LASIK satisfaction. LASIK Newswire Web site. http://www.lasiknewswire.com/2009/12/the-truth-behind-lasik-satisfaction.html. Updated December 13, 2009. Accessed January 19, 2015.

Chapter 10

For Cataract Patients With Astigmatism
Toric Intraocular Lenses

IN THE BEGINNING WAS SIR HAROLD

Almost any book or book chapter on intraocular lenses (IOLs) probably needs to start with the words "Sir Harold Ridley." As most ophthalmologists know, Ridley implanted the first IOL, made of a hard polymer called polymethylmethacrylate (PMMA). During World War II, Ridley treated Royal Air Force pilots and noticed that when splinters of PMMA from aircraft cockpit canopies became lodged in their eyes, there was no rejection response as happens with glass splinters. Ridley commissioned the Rayner Company, of Brighton & Hove, East Sussex, to manufacture an IOL using PMMA (brand name Perspex). He implanted the first of these lenses on November 29, 1949, at St. Thomas Hospital.[1,2] The Rayner Company continues to manufacture and market small-incision IOLs today.[2]

IOLs remained largely a European phenomenon until arriving in the United States later in the 1950s, where their use grew through the 1960s and 1970s (see Figure 10-1). The first IOL implanted in the United States was a Ridley-Rayner lens, in a procedure performed in 1957 at Wills Eye Hospital, Philadelphia.[3] I converted to extracapsular cataract extraction in 1982, implanting Shearing-style IOLs in the posterior chamber. For a number of reasons, not the least of which was the imminent availability of small-incision IOLs, I converted from extracapsular cataract extraction to phacoemulsification (phaco) in 1987, which makes me an early adopter of phaco in Australia (see Sidebar 10-1). In the early 1980s, only 10% of eye surgeons performed phaco, escalating to 95% by 1995. Obviously, phaco allowed surgeons to take advantage of the small incision afforded by foldable IOLs[1] with better control of the astigmatism change induced by the surgery.

TORIC IOLS:
LEADING THE WAY INTO THE 21ST CENTURY

Toric IOLs are considered a "premium" lens in the United States, for which Medicare, Medicaid, and most medical insurance plans require beneficiaries to pay an additional amount out of pocket (this also applies to aspheric, bifocal, multifocal, and

Alpins N. *Practical Astigmatism:
Planning and Analysis* (pp 77-85).
© 2018 SLACK Incorporated.

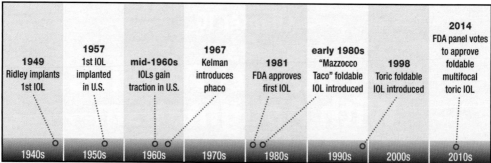

Figure 10-1. The first IOLs were made of a rigid plastic, PMMA, which required a 5-mm to 7-mm incision for insertion.[4] Although Charles Kelman introduced phacoemulsification in 1967, prior to the introduction of foldable IOLs in the mid-1980s, extracapsular cataract extraction (ECCE) was the norm.[1] In conjunction with ECCE, surgeons who wished to correct astigmatism during cataract/IOL surgery would use incision placement, selective suture removal, and/or astigmatic incisional keratotomies.[4] Surgeons quickly converted from ECCE to phacoemulsification during the 1980s in order to take advantage of the small incision afforded by foldable IOLs.[1] Since the introduction of foldable toric IOLs in the late 1990s,[4] more and more surgeons are using foldable toric IOLs for patients with "visually significant" levels of astigmatism, usually thought to be about 1 D to 1.5 D of cylinder or greater. The US Food and Drug Administration (FDA) approved an accommodating foldable IOL in 2013[4]; the FDA Ophthalmic Devices Panel voted to approve a foldable multifocal toric IOL in late 2014.[5] Abbreviations: FDA, Food and Drug Administration; IOL, intraocular lens; PMMA, polymethylmethacrylate.

accommodating IOLs, or combinations thereof).[4] Most carriers cover the full cost of standard small-incision IOLs, and it is possible at some point, that features now considered premium will come to be regarded as standard, with a cost that is fully covered. In the days when a limited variety of IOLs were approved and available, the choice of IOL was more or less up to the surgeon. Today, that choice requires a conversation with the cataract patient, who has the chance to participate in the decision by considering the relative cost, risks, and benefits of currently available IOLs.[4]

A limited selection of small-incision toric IOLs are approved for use in the United States[6]; many other designs and brands are available elsewhere in the world.[7] Despite the additional cost to US patients, however, the use of toric IOLs appears to be on the rise. Since 2000, investigators also appear to have a growing interest in toric IOLs (see Figure 10-2).

Studies show that 15% to 29% of patients with cataracts have > 1.5 D of refractive astigmatism.[8,9] What percentage of patients have similar degrees of corneal astigmatism? In my practice, 17% of patients with cataract have more than 1.50 D of corneal astigmatism preoperatively (N = > 7000 eyes).

The increasing use of toric IOLs may be related to the additional cost and risk of a secondary procedure for patients with monofocal IOLs who later decide they would like to have better, uncorrected vision. The options for these patients include incisional astigmatic keratotomy, laser in situ keratomileusis (LASIK), or lifetime use of contact lenses or spectacles in order to achieve satisfactory vision.[4,10,11]

This is not to say that toric IOLs have no risks. It is simply that surgeons and their patients who understand these risks often appear to come down on the benefit side of the risk-benefit ratio, and that decision appears to be a growing trend.

Sidebar 10-1
The Road to the Alpins Method Ran Through Phaco

I first met Howard Gimbel, of Calgary, Alberta, Canada, in 1986 "under the banyan tree" at the Royal Hawaiian Eye Meeting in Maui. With his tutelage and encouragement, I began a conversion from extracapsular cataract extraction to phacoemulsification in May 1987, modeling every detail of my approach after Howard's, including his divide-and-conquer technique and brilliant innovation, capsulorrhexis capsulotomy that came a little later. Thanks mainly to Howard, I was one of the first Australian surgeons to offer small-incision cataract surgery, and the first in Melbourne, Victoria.

In 1993, Howard invited me to speak at his Canadian Rockies symposium. He invited me to speak again in 1994, which was the 10th and final Canadian Rockies symposium. I had published my first paper on the Alpins Method by then, and Howard was one of the first ophthalmologists to ask me for further details on Vector Planning, which I had already developed and was using, but was not published until 1997. In 1994, Howard announced at a large VisX meeting in San Francisco that he was going to be using the ASSORT program, which is a comprehensive ophthalmic program that includes the Alpins Method of astigmatism analysis by refractive and corneal parameters. One can only admire him for his forward thinking and his trust in my concepts at such an early stage of their popularization. His encouragement was most heartening.

I met Steven Siepser, of Wayne, Pennsylvania, at the Aspen meeting in 1991, after which he visited me in Melbourne later that year, and helped to get me invited as a speaker at Aspen the following year (1992). I had been doing phaco for a number of years by that time, and I performed vector analyses on the various incisions I used. To prepare for that meeting, I gathered my data together and hired a computer programmer, John Carragher, to help in the graphic presentation of my findings. My preparations for that meeting comprised the seminal incentive in the development of the Alpins Method.

PLANNING AND MEASUREMENT

An important component to obtaining good visual outcomes after toric IOL implantation begins with accurate measurement of preoperative corneal astigmatism (magnitude and orientation). Instruments used to measure corneal astigmatism include topography, IOL Master (Carl Zeiss Meditec), Lenstar (Haag-Streit), manual keratometry, and tomography (including the posterior cornea). Many clinicians use more than one of these approaches to determine the final corneal astigmatism value on which to base toric IOL selection.

All of the previously-mentioned devices determine corneal astigmatism based on a narrow section of the cornea. For example, the simulated keratometry from topography is based on one Placido ring. A calculation we call corneal topographic astigmatism (CorT) uses data acquired from the entire cornea to obtain a vectorial mean. In cases where the posterior cornea is also measured, we calculate what we call CorT total, which takes into account the posterior cornea (see Chapter 12 for a full discussion of CorT and CorT total).

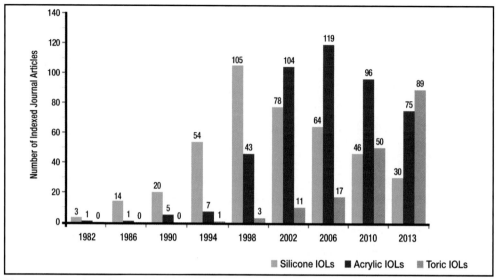

Figure 10-2. PubMed was searched for journal articles published in the years shown. Three different searches were conducted: (1) "yearpub + silicone + intraocular + lens"; (2) "yearpub + acrylic + intraocular + lens"; and (3) "yearpub + toric + intraocular + lens." Such searches would not capture all possible candidate articles, but were meant only to reveal the trends, which are apparent in the graph. Abbreviations: IOL, intraocular lens; yearpub, year of publication.

The next step in obtaining optimal visual outcomes with toric IOLs is to select an accurate calculator. The toric IOL calculator should consider the following:
1. Axial length of the eye
2. Refractive index of the instrument used to measure the preoperative corneal astigmatism
3. Personalized IOL constants to accurately calculate the effective lens position
4. Adjustment of the IOL toricity for the spherical component of the IOL when converting from IOL plane to corneal plane
5. Allowing for the flattening effect of the main phaco incision when determining the amount and orientation of the corneal astigmatism that is being neutralized

All these factors are included in the ASSORT Toric IOL Calculator (ASSORT [Alpins Statistical System for Ophthalmic Refractive surgery Techniques]), available free at www.assort.com (see Figure 10-3). This and other ASSORT programs are described in greater detail in Chapter 24. Many of the corporate toric IOL calculators available at manufacturers' respective websites are missing one or more of the essential components described above.

Postoperatively, the corneal astigmatism should once again be measured to determine if the phaco incision performed as expected, particularly if the refractive cylinder obtained is unexpected. Furthermore, we prefer using the same device and even the same technician postoperatively, as well as preoperatively.

Measuring corneal astigmatism accurately by one or several devices is key to good toric IOL outcomes. Measurements should be repeatable, and the surgeon should factor in the contribution of the posterior cornea to the total corneal astigmatism.[10,12] This brings the corneal astigmatism closer to the total astigmatism of the eye as measured by manifest refractive cylinder.

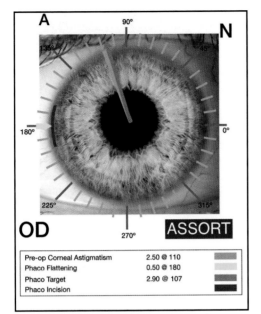 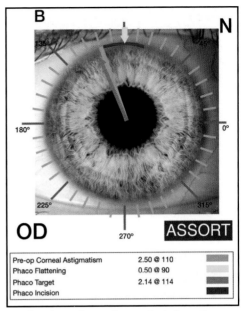

Figure 10-3. ASSORT (www.assort.com) incorporates active dynamics to demonstrate how the preoperative corneal astigmatism changes in magnitude and orientation depending on the position and amount of flattening effect of the phaco incision. The phaco incision is displayed at 180° (A) and 90° (B), in each case changing the preoperative magnitude and orientation by displacing the astigmatism away from it.

MATERIALS, DIMENSIONS, AND POWERS

Toric IOLs available in the United States are made of both silicone and acrylic materials (see Figure 10-4). In general, silicone toric IOLs require a slightly wider incision than acrylic toric IOLs due to plate-haptic design—3 mm as compared to 2.2 mm, respectively.[13] Toric IOLs requiring a "microincision" of < 2 mm have been studied[14,15] and likely will gain widespread availability.

The silicone plate-haptic designs are available with two different overall lengths: 10.8 mm and 11.2 mm. Most acrylic lens styles have 6-mm optics. In the United States, spherical powers range from 0 D to 34 D; cylinder powers at the IOL plane range from 1 D to 9 D. Outside the United States, toric IOLs can be customized and are available from -30 D to +45 D for sphere and +0.25 D to +30 D for cylinder.

CLINICAL TRIAL RESULTS

A review of toric IOL studies by Sinha et al[16] highlights the excellent visual acuity results seen in patients receiving a toric IOL, with both corrected and uncorrected distance visual acuities of 20/40 or better attained by 40% to 99% of patients depending on the study, and better visual acuity outcomes than monofocal IOLs in all studies that included a control group having similar levels of preoperative astigmatism. Axis misalignments of toric IOLs > 5° are uncommon—typically in the single-digit percentages.

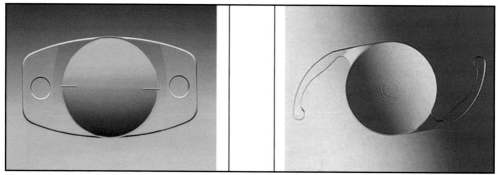

Figure 10-4. Two common styles of toric IOL, made of silicone (left) and acrylic (right) polymers. The silicone plate-haptic design should not be implanted in a compromised capsular bag, and may be more prone to postoperative rotation.

The US FDA-approved labeling for one acrylic toric IOL includes the following results[17]:

- 94% of patients with uncorrected distance vision of 20/40 or better
- Improved contrast sensitivity in low light
- Significant reduction in both spherical and total higher-order aberrations
- Improved functional vision in adverse conditions such as night driving, glare, and fog

One controlled study included patients with similar degrees of preoperative astigmatism, randomly assigned to groups receiving a toric IOL or a monofocal IOL.[11] In addition to significantly better visual results, patients receiving a toric IOL enjoyed significantly better scores in a validated quality-of-life instrument which included clarity of vision, far vision, glare and satisfaction with correction (Table 10-1).

MISALIGNMENT AND OTHER ERRORS

Decreased vision due to a toric IOL rotating out of alignment or not placed in the most effective orientation are not uncommon and a second procedure may be needed to realign the IOL, replace the IOL, or perform excimer laser surgery.[4,10,12] Surgical planning and treatment approaches for these "refractive surprises" are described in Chapter 11.

The common wisdom is that a 15° misalignment of a toric IOL causes up to a 45% loss of effect.[12] Some surgeons have reported a 33% loss of toric correction with an off-axis placement of 10°, or about 3% off axis per degree.[18] These reports reflect a scalar analysis comparing postoperative refractive cylinder to preoperative corneal astigmatism. Vectorial analysis, readily performed with ASSORT, shows that a misalignment of 15° causes only a 13.4% loss of effect.[12,19]

The more "forgiving" nature of toric IOL off-axis placement was confirmed by an optoelectronic bench test,[20] performed by Daniele Tognetto, MD. The bench study, reported in *Ocular Surgery News* in 2014, showed that, although the common wisdom holds that off-axis placement of 30° induces the loss of the entire cylindrical correction, the total loss of toric effect does not occur until a 45° misalignment is reached.

Table 10-1

Scores for the National Eye Institute Refractive Error Quality-of-Life Instrument—42 Questionnaire, Administered 3 Months After IOL Implantation

	Astigmatic Control Group (n=40 eyes) Receiving Monofocal IOL	Astigmatic Group (n=40 eyes) Receiving Toric IOL	*P* Value
Clarity of vision	78.10 ± 12.39	95.17 ± 7.47	< .001
Far vision	61.5 ± 20.7	79.4 ± 18.3	.021
Glare	79.5 ± 11.6	89.6 ± 12.3	.038
Satisfaction with correction	78.2 ± 14.0	97.8 ± 6.5	.001

Reprinted with permission from Mencucci R, Giordano C, Favuzza E, Gicquel J-J, Spadea L, Menchini U. Astigmatism correction with toric intraocular lenses. *Br J Ophthalmol*. 2013;97(5):578-582.

It is important to understand the context in which the misalignment of a toric IOL and its outcome is mentioned. Some studies report the change in manifest refractive cylinder as a result of toric IOL rotation; others calculate the loss in terms of neutralizing the corneal astigmatism as a result of misalignment. The calculation for each scenario may be correct, but the parameters and analysis type should be considered.

Some common errors reported when implanting toric IOLs include[18]:
- Inaccurate preoperative measurements.
- Omitting axial length, device refractive index, and optimized lens constants.
- Incorrect preoperative marking of reference points on the cornea.
- Incorrect alignment of the toric IOL.
- Failure to consider the impact of surgically induced astigmatism vector (SIA).
- Incorrect toricity of the IOL at the corneal plane.
- Failure to factor in the patient's posterior corneal power.
- Measurement variability.

With time, experience, and better planning, cataract surgeons will find these problems to be less and less common.

THE ALPINS METHOD AND TORIC IOLS IN THE LITERATURE

A toric IOL analysis has an important difference from a refractive or corneal vectorial analysis: It is a hybrid analysis that determines the SIA refractive effect of the toric implant by comparing the postoperative refractive cylinder to the preoperative phaco-adjusted corneal astigmatism.

A number of toric IOL studies have utilized the Alpins Method in one way or another.[10,14,15,21-28] These authors utilized whichever indices of the Alpins Method they thought relevant to their studies. The indices they used—such as difference vector, angle of error, correction index, and index of success—provide a reliable yardstick to compare their clinical results to each other and other modes of astigmatism correction. Even a cursory review instills the sense that apples are finally being compared to apples. Additionally, the *Journal of Refractive Surgery* is defining Alpins Method-related standard graphs for reporting toric IOL studies.[29,30] For me, it is a wholly gratifying experience.

References

1. Boyle EL. Foldable IOLs ushered in new cataract and refractive paradigm. *Ocular Surgery News*. June 1, 2007.
2. Apple DJ, Sims J. Harold Ridley and the Invention of the Intraocular Lens. Rayner Web site. http://www.rayner.com/skin/frontend/mtcolias/default/pdf/Invention_of_the_IOL.pdf. Accessed June 15, 2017.
3. Letocha CE, Pavlin CJ. Follow-up of 3 patients with Ridley intraocular lens implantation. *J Cataract Refract Surg*. 1999;25(4):587-591.
4. Segre L, Haddrill M. Intraocular lenses (IOLs): including premium, toric and aspheric designs. AllAboutVision com Web site. http://www.allaboutvision.com/conditions/iols.htm. Accessed November 18, 2014.
5. FDA panel recommends premarket approval application for AcrySof IQ ReSTOR multifocal toric IOL. Ocular Surgery News Web site. http://www.healio.com/ophthalmology/regulatory-legislative/news/online/%7Ba6a271c3d-a34b-4a4e-9d1b-25517963ed77%7D/fda-panel-recommends-premarket-approval-application-for-acrysof-iq-restor-multifocal-toric-iol. Accessed November 18, 2014.
6. Matossian C. Toric IOL properties. Eyeworld Web Site. http://www.eyeworld.org/article-toric-iol-properties. Accessed November 20, 2014.
7. Chang JSM, Dewey S, Jackson MA, Packer M, Stonecipher KG. Update on the premium IOL markets in the United States and Asia. Cataract & Refractive Surgery Today Web site. http://bmctoday.net/crstodayeurope/2013/01/article.asp?f=update-on-the-premium-iol-markets-in-the-united-states-and-asia. Accessed November 20, 2014.
8. Hoffer KJ. Biometry of 7,500 cataractous eyes. *Am J Ophthalmol*. 1980;90(3):360-368.
9. Ninn-Pedersen K, Stenevi U, Ehinger B. Cataract patients in a defined Swedish population 1986-1990. II. Preoperative observations. *Acta Ophthalmol (Copenh)*. 1994;72(1):10-15.
10. Alpins N, Ong JK, Stamatelatos G. Refractive surprise after toric intraocular lens implantation: graph analysis. *J Cataract Refract Surg*. 2014;40(2):283-294.
11. Mencucci R, Giordano C, Favuzza E, Gicquel J-J, Spadea L, Menchini U. Astigmatism correction with toric intraocular lenses. *Br J Ophthalmol*. 2013;97(5):578-582.
12. Alpins N, Stamatelatos G. Correcting refractive surprises after toric IOL implantation. *Cataract & Refractive Surgery Today Europe*. 2014:20-22.
13. Patel AS, Feldman BH, Fajardo D, Stelzner SK, Griffiths D, WikiWorks Team. Toric IOLs. American Academy of Ophthalmology Web site. http://eyewiki.aao.org/Toric_IOLs. Accessed November 18, 2014.
14. Mojzis P, Pinero DP, Studeny P, et al. Comparative analysis of clinical outcomes obtained with a new diffractive multifocal toric intraocular lens implanted through two types of corneal incision. *J Refract Surg*. 2011;27(9):648-657.
15. Alio JL, Agdeppa MC, Pongo VC, El KB. Microincision cataract surgery with toric intraocular lens implantation for correcting moderate and high astigmatism: pilot study. *J Cataract Refract Surg*. 2010;36(1):44-52.

16. Sinha R, Shekhar H, Tinwala S, Rathi A, Titiyal JS. Toric intraocular lenses: a review. *J Clin Ophthalmol Res.* 2013;1:193-196.

17. Recognize both. Recommend AcrySof IQ toric IOL [brochure]. Alcon Web site. https://www.myalcon.com/products/surgical/docs/surgeon_brochure.pdf. Accessed November 21, 2014.

18. Roach L. Toric IOLs: four options for addressing residual astigmatism. American Academy of Ophthalmology Web site. http://www.aao.org/publications/eyenet/201204/cataract.cfm. Accessed November 21, 2014.

19. Alpins NA. Vector analysis of astigmatism changes by flattening, steepening, and torque. *J Cataract Refract Surg.* 1997;23(10):1503-1514.

20. Tognetto D, Rinaldi S, Bauci F, et al. Quality of images with toric intraocular lenses. *J Cataract Refract Surg.* In press.

21. Alio JL, Pinero DP, Tomas J, Aleson A. Vector analysis of astigmatic changes after cataract surgery with toric intraocular lens implantation. *J Cataract Refract Surg.* 2011;37(6):1038-1049.

22. Alio JL, Pinero DP, Tomas J, Plaza AB. Vector analysis of astigmatic changes after cataract surgery with implantation of a new toric multifocal intraocular lens. *J Cataract Refract Surg.* 2011;37(7):1217-1229.

23. Bellucci R, Bauer NJ, Daya SM et al. Visual acuity and refraction with a diffractive multifocal toric intraocular lens. *J Cataract Refract Surg.* 2013;39(10):1507-1518.

24. Chassain C. [Evaluation of visual performance after implantation of a double C-Loop toric intraocular lens]. *J Fr Ophtalmol.* 2014;37(7):507-513.

25. Freitas GO, Boteon JE, Carvalho MJ, Pinto RM. Treatment of astigmatism during phacoemulsification. *Arq Bras Oftalmol.* 2014;77(1):40-46.

26. Hoffmann PC, Auel S, Hutz WW. Results of higher power toric intraocular lens implantation. *J Cataract Refract Surg.* 2011;37(8):1411-1418.

27. Humbert G, Colin J, Touboul D. [AcrySof(R) Toric (SN60T) intraocular lens implantation: refractive predictibility and aberrometric impact of decentration]. *J Fr Ophtalmol.* 2013;36(4):352-361.

28. Visser N, Berendschot TT, Bauer NJ, Nuijts RM. Vector analysis of corneal and refractive astigmatism changes following toric pseudophakic and toric phakic IOL implantation. *Invest Ophthalmol Vis Sci.* 2012;53(4):1865-1873.

29. Reinstein DZ, Randleman JB, Archer TJ, et al. JRS standard for reporting outcomes of intraocular lens based refractive surgery. *J Refract Surg.* 2017;33(4):218-222.

30. Reinstein DZ, Archer TJ, Srinivasan S, et al. Standard for reporting refractive outcomes of intraocular lens-based refractive surgery. *J Cataract Refract Surg.* 2017;43(4):435-439.

Chapter 11

Analysis and Management of "Refractive Surprises" After Toric Intraocular Lens Implantation

TORIC INTRAOCULAR LENS COMPLICATES REFRACTIVE ANALYSIS

Cataract surgeons usually select the power of an intraocular lens (IOL) with the aim to achieve emmetropia. Unfortunately, even when the latest devices and planning software are used, postoperative refractive surprises inevitably occur. The situation becomes much more complicated when a toric IOL has been implanted because the IOL's orientation, cylinder power, and spherical power all must be considered.

Toric IOLs have been shown to provide good visual acuity (VA) and rotational stability. Table 11-1 shows VA and rotational stability results in a variety of clinical studies where both types of outcomes were measured and reported.

Perhaps contributing to the good VA results is the fact that the loss of astigmatic effect due to toric IOL misalignment is often overstated. The "common wisdom" is that a 15° misalignment results in a loss of effect of 45% (based on a scalar comparison of astigmatism magnitudes postoperatively vs preoperatively). Vectorial calculation indicates that a 15° misalignment causes a 13.4% loss of effect[1] (Figure 11-1).

In another study employing optoelectronic bench testing, a misalignment up to 5° caused a decrease of 7% in image definition; at 15°, the loss was about 20%; at 25°, the loss was 40%; and at 45°, image definition degraded by more than 50%—to a point where the image obtained was comparable to one having no cylindrical correction.[2]

ACCURACY: A KEY ELEMENT IN OUTCOMES

Accuracy is a key ingredient of the many steps in planning and implanting a toric IOL. The accuracy—and repeatability—of devices that provide measures of axial length and corneal astigmatism is a fundamental concern. The surgeon should use a personalized IOL constant and know the flattening effect of the surgically induced astigmatism vector (SIA) rather than the whole SIA (as is suggested by some authors) associated with his or her preferred phaco incision (Sidebar 11-1); see Chapter 10 for additional informa-

Alpins N. *Practical Astigmatism:
Planning and Analysis* (pp 87-93).
© 2018 SLACK Incorporated.

Table 11-1
Rotational Stability and Visual Acuity Results of Toric Intraocular Lenses in Various Published Clinical Studies

Study	N/n	Rotational Stability Results	Visual Acuity Results
Alió et al, 2010[3]	21 eyes in 12 patients implanted with toric IOLs through a microincision (< 2 mm)	At 3 months, mean IOL axis rotation was -1.75° ± 2.93°; rotation was ≤ 10° in all eyes.	At 3 months, UDVA 20/40 or better in 76.1%; BCDVA 20/30 or better in 85.7%.
Holland et al, 2010[4]	Toric IOL, n = 256; control IOL, n = 261	Mean rotation < 4° (range, 0°–20°) in toric IOL group.	BCDVA ≥ 20/20 in 77.7% of toric IOL group vs 69.2% of control IOL group 1 year postop. UDVA 20/20 or better was 40.7% in toric IOL group vs 19.4% in control IOL group (*P* < .05).
Ahmed et al, 2010[5]	Bilateral toric IOLs in 117 patients (234 eyes)	At 6 months, IOL alignment was within ±5° in 91% of eyes and within ±10° in 99%.	Binocular UDVA 20/40 or better in 99% and 20/20 or better in 63% of patients.
Mendicute et al, 2008[6]	30 eyes in 15 consecutive patients	Mean toric IOL rotation was 3.63° ± 3.11°, with rotation < 10° in 96.7% of eyes.	UDVA 20/40 or better in 93.3% of eyes; 20/25 or better in 66.6%. All eyes achieved 20/25 or better BCDVA.
De Silva et al, 2006[7]	21 eyes of 14 consecutive patients	No IOL rotated more than 5° during the 6-month follow-up.	At 6 months, 79% had UDVA of 20/35 or better.
Shimizu et al, 1994[8]	2-D toric IOLs (n=26) and 3-D toric IOLs (n=21)	3-D toric IOLs resulted in better VA than 2-D toric IOLs with axis shifts < 30°. A negative effect occurred in some eyes in which IOLs rotated ≥ 30°. The maximum acceptable axis shift appeared to be < 30°.	BCDVA 3 months postoperatively was 20/25 or better in 77% of eyes.

Abbreviations: BCDVA, best corrected distance visual acuity; UDVA, uncorrected distance visual acuity; VA, visual acuity.

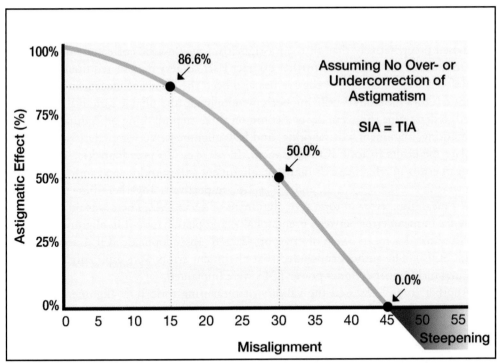

Figure 11-1. The relationship between the misalignment of a toric IOL and reduction of astigmatic effect is not linear, but sigmoidal/trigonometric. A 30° misalignment is necessary for astigmatic effect to be degraded 50%; a 15° misalignment reduces astigmatic effect only about 13%. The figure assumes that, in this patient, SIA equals TIA (there is no over- or undercorrection). (Reprinted with permission from Alpins N, Stamatelatos G. Correcting refractive surprises after toric IOL implantation. *CRST Europe.* 2014:20-22.)

Sidebar 11-1
Implanting a Toric IOL? Know Your Flattening Effect!

The flattening effect (FE) quantifies the effect of an incision. In the case of cataract surgery, surgeons should know the historical FE of their preferred incision, particularly when implanting toric IOLs, as the FE can alter both the power and orientation of the toric IOL that is selected.

The FE is a more accurate parameter than the SIA, as it is represents the astigmatic change occurring at the meridian of the incision, whereas the SIA is calculated as the total change between the preoperative and postoperative astigmatism, wherever the orientation may be.

tion on toric IOLs. Importantly, an existing or longstanding ocular residual astigmatism (ORA) may not be evident due to the presence of the cataract[9,10]; thus, patients should be advised preoperatively that all their astigmatism may not be corrected and the need for a rotation of the implant or further excimer laser surgery may be required.

Reference axis marking of the eye has also been the source of inaccurate alignment of a toric IOL. One study[11] utilizing both pseudophakic and phakic toric IOLs was conducted to determine the accuracy of a common three-step marking procedure: reference axis marking, alignment axis marking, and IOL alignment. Vector analysis was used to calculate the errors in toric IOL alignment. In 40 eyes (26 pseudophakic, 14 phakic), the mean errors in reference axis marking, alignment axis marking, and toric IOL alignment were 2.4° ± 0.8°, 3.3° ± 2°, and 2.6° ± 2.6°, respectively. Together, these three errors led to a mean total error in toric IOL alignment of 4.9° ± 2.1°. There was no significant difference in mean error between pseudophakic and phakic toric IOL alignment. Vector analysis showed a mean angle of error of –2° ± 8° (pseudophakic IOLs) and 6° ± 14° (phakic IOLs). The authors concluded that alignment errors were especially relevant in cases in which higher-cylinder-power IOLs were implanted.

Another study[12] assessed the validity of measuring toric IOL alignment with the internal optical-path-difference (OPD) map of a corneal analyzer system vs a slit lamp. An internal OPD map is a wavefront map plotting the refractive effect of all the aberrations of the eye except the front corneal surface (basically, the ORA). In this retrospective study, the toric IOL axis was measured 3 weeks postoperatively by rotating the slit lamp beam to align with the IOL axis indicator marks and using the internal OPD map on a corneal analyzer system. The mean IOL misalignment measured by slit lamp was 2.55° ± 2.76° and by the internal map, 2.65° ± 1.98°. The correlation between the two methods was highly significant ($P < .001$). The authors concluded that both the refractive power/corneal analyzer system and slit lamp observation were reliable and predictable methods of assessing toric IOL alignment.

CALCULATING THE PLAN FOR TORIC IOL IMPLANTATION

For a number of reasons, a toric IOL can end up in an axial orientation different from what was intended, becoming misaligned either during surgery or at some point after implantation.[13,14] Even when a toric IOL has the correct power and orientation, an astigmatic refractive surprise is possible.

As noted in Chapter 10, the phaco incision itself induces an astigmatic effect—one that should be taken into consideration in planning the implantation of a toric IOL. The ASSORT Toric IOL Calculator (ASSORT [Alpins Statistical System for Ophthalmic Refractive surgery Techniques]), available free at www.assort.com, enables consideration of this variable as well as a number of others involved in the planning of toric IOL implantation and interventions to correct any postoperative refractive surprises.

As cataract surgeons are well aware, the effective lens position is best calculated using the surgeon's personalized IOL constants. ASSORT allows the entry of the SRK/T A-constant, the Holladay surgeon factor, the Hoffer Q pseudophakic anterior chamber depth (ACD), and the Haigis formula, which uses ACD1 (Figure 11-2).

ASSORT displays the most suitable IOLs (among all toric IOLs available worldwide

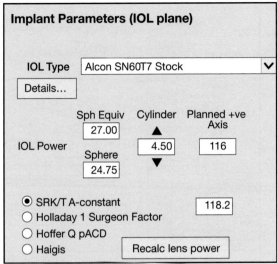

Implant Parameters (IOL plane)

IOL Type: Alcon SN60T7 Stock

Details...

IOL Power

Sph Equiv 27.00

Cylinder 4.50

Planned +ve Axis 116

Sphere 24.75

◉ SRK/T A-constant 118.2
○ Holladay 1 Surgeon Factor
○ Hoffer Q pACD
○ Haigis   Recalc lens power

Figure 11-2. The effective lens position is accurately calculated using the surgeon's personalized IOL constants. The ability to select any toric IOL currently manufactured worldwide is a unique feature of ASSORT. This offers the advantage of being able to compare different IOLs for each case without having to go to several manufacturers' websites, where there is a variability in calculation method and accuracy.

at this writing) according to the preoperative parameters that are entered, together with the expected postoperative spherocylindrical refraction in positive- or negative-cylinder format. The user has the ability to paste this content into an email and order the IOL from his or her local representative.

CALCULATING THE SOLUTION TO THE REFRACTIVE SURPRISE

ASSORT enables the practitioner to solve for postoperative refractive surprises, which occur when the patient has some unexpected cylinder remaining in his or her refraction. To do this, the user enters the postoperative axis of the IOL and the postoperative spherocylindrical refraction. The display (Figure 11-3) shows the amount and direction of IOL rotation required to obtain the minimum refractive cylinder for the implanted toric IOL.

In some cases, the amount of cylinder that can be reduced by IOL rotation is not sufficient to fully correct the remaining astigmatism. This is the case when the calculations produce a shallow sigmoidal curve. In that case, the Alpins Method of astigmatism analysis, which is programmed into the online calculator, advises the user as to whether IOL exchange or laser in situ keratomileusis (LASIK) may be the better option to address the remaining error (Figure 11-4). If the magnitude of error is > 1 D, then the toric power of the IOL is incorrect and an IOL exchange or LASIK may be indicated.

ASSORT is divided into two modules so that the surgeon can go right into the postoperative refractive surprises module without having to enter all the preoperative data. With ASSORT, we have tried to make planning and analyses of toric IOLs as transparent as possible to allow surgeons to improve their astigmatic outcomes with toric implants. As more manufacturers develop toric IOLs, their specifications will be added to the ASSORT calculator selection.

Figure 11-3. This screen shows the amount and direction of rotation of the toric intraocular lens required to minimize refractive cylinder. Note that corneal refractive index, axial length, optimized lens constants, and implant sphere are included in the calculation.

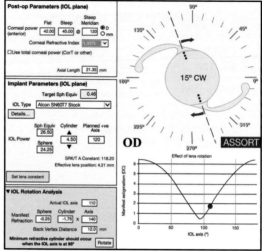

Figure 11-4. The Alpins Method of astigmatism analysis determines the correction index and magnitude of error, indicating if the correct powered toricity of the intraocular lens has been selected.

Alpins Method			
SIA	4.44	Ax	37
TIA	3.36	Ax	30
Difference Vector	1.45	Ax	145
Correction Index	1.32		
Index of Success	0.43		
Magnitude of Error	1.09		
Angle of Error	7 (CCW)		

SUMMARY OF THE ASSORT CALCULATOR

- Calculations for the most appropriate toric IOL should take into account the effect of the phaco incision, the axial length of the eye, the refractive index of the instrument used to measure the preoperative corneal astigmatism, the surgeon's personalized IOL constant, and the spherical component of the IOL, as the toric power at the corneal plane will vary depending on the spherical power. Whatever calculator is used when deciding how much rotation might be required, it should allow the entry of all these variables (not all calculators do so).
- With the ASSORT Toric IOL Calculator, toric implants from all manufacturers can be compared to see which is best for a particular patient.
- A unique feature of ASSORT software is the ability to solve for postoperative refractive surprises, which occur when the patient has some unexpected cylinder remaining in his or her refraction.

REFERENCES

1. Alpins N, Stamatelatos G. Correcting refractive surprises after toric IOL implantation. *Cataract & Refractive Surgery Today Europe.* 2014:20-22.

2. Tognetto D, Rinaldi S, Bauci F, et al. Quality of images with toric intraocular lenses. *J Cataract Refract Surg.* In press.

3. Alio JL, Agdeppa MC, Pongo VC, El KB. Microincision cataract surgery with toric intraocular lens implantation for correcting moderate and high astigmatism: pilot study. *J Cataract Refract Surg.* 2010;36(1):44-52.

4. Holland E, Lane S, Horn JD, Ernest P, Arleo R, Miller KM. The AcrySof Toric intraocular lens in subjects with cataracts and corneal astigmatism: a randomized, subject-masked, parallel-group, 1-year study. *Ophthalmology.* 2010;117(11):2104-2111.

5. Ahmed II, Rocha G, Slomovic AR, et al. Visual function and patient experience after bilateral implantation of toric intraocular lenses. *J Cataract Refract Surg.* 2010;36(4):609-616.

6. Mendicute J, Irigoyen C, Aramberri J, Ondarra A, Montes-Mico R. Foldable toric intraocular lens for astigmatism correction in cataract patients. *J Cataract Refract Surg.* 2008;34(4):601-607.

7. De Silva DJ, Ramkissoon YD, Bloom PA. Evaluation of a toric intraocular lens with a Z-haptic. *J Cataract Refract Surg.* 2006;32(9):1492-1498.

8. Shimizu K, Misawa A, Suzuki Y. Toric intraocular lenses: correcting astigmatism while controlling axis shift. *J Cataract Refract Surg.* 1994;20(5):523-526.

9. Alpins NA. New method of targeting vectors to treat astigmatism. *J Cataract Refract Surg.* 1997;23(1):65-75.

10. Koch DD, Ali SF, Weikert MP, Shirayama M, Jenkins R, Wang L. Contribution of posterior corneal astigmatism to total corneal astigmatism. *J Cataract Refract Surg.* 2012;38(12):2080-2087.

11. Visser N, Berendschot TT, Bauer NJ, Jurich J, Kersting O, Nuijts RM. Accuracy of toric intraocular lens implantation in cataract and refractive surgery. *J Cataract Refract Surg.* 2011;37(8):1394-1402.

12. Carey PJ, Leccisotti A, McGilligan VE, Goodall EA, Moore CB. Assessment of toric intraocular lens alignment by a refractive power/corneal analyzer system and slitlamp observation. *J Cataract Refract Surg.* 2010;36(2):222-229.

13. Patel CK, Ormonde S, Rosen PH, Bron AJ. Postoperative intraocular lens rotation: a randomized comparison of plate and loop haptic implants. *Ophthalmology.* 1999;106(11):2190-2195.

14. Shah GD, Praveen MR, Vasavada AR, Vasavada VA, Rampal G, Shastry LR. Rotational stability of a toric intraocular lens: influence of axial length and alignment in the capsular bag. *J Cataract Refract Surg.* 2012;38(1):54-59.

Chapter 12

Corneal Topographic Astigmatism
A Measure of Anterior and Total Corneal Power

CORNEAL TOPOGRAPHIC ASTIGMATISM AND BEYOND: CORNEAL TOPOGRAPHIC ASTIGMATISM TOTAL

Evolution of the Anterior Picture

In the beginning, there was Hermann von Helmholtz, who published his design for a keratometer, which he called an ophthalmometer, in the mid-19th century.[1,2] It came to pass in the mid-1960s that the term photokeratoscopy began to appear in the literature,[3,4] followed about 25 years later with a technique called computer-assisted video keratography or corneal topography. The anterior corneal astigmatism revealed by this image manipulation, quantified as simulated keratometry (SimK),[5] demonstrated equivalence with the prevailing technology, manual keratometry.

And so SimK became widely used by cataract and refractive surgeons. In 2012, we introduced a term called corneal topographic astigmatism (CorT),[6] which correlates with manifest refractive cylinder more closely than SimK for reasons that include the acquisition of all data captured across the cornea (Figure 12-1).

SimK is a measurement calculated by corneal topography instruments and displayed with corneal topography maps. As shown in Figure 12-1, SimK is based on corneal astigmatism around the 3-mm zone. In contrast, CorT is based on measured data across a wide annular region on the cornea, gathered from all visible Placido rings.[6]

In addition to SimK, CorT is also more closely aligned to the manifest refractive cylinder than manual keratometry, corneal wavefront measurement, and paraxial curvature matching. Since CorT—a summated vector mean of astigmatism values from all complete, visible Placido rings—does a better job in approaching the magnitude and axis of manifest refractive cylinder than the other commonly used measures of corneal astigmatism, the calculated ocular residual astigmatism (ORA)—that is, the vectorial difference between refractive and corneal astigmatism as described in Chapter 9—is less in these eyes using CorT, both in magnitude and variability, than it would be with the other common methods studied[6] (Figure 12-2).

Alpins N. *Practical Astigmatism: Planning and Analysis* (pp 95-104).

Figure 12-1. (A) SimK is calculated using a single Placido ring. (B) CorT utilizes all valid data. (C) The CorT is closer in magnitude and orientation to the manifest refractive cylinder than SimK.[7] CorT is also closer to refractive cylinder than corneal wavefront and paraxial curvature matching.[6] Abbreviations: CorT, corneal topographic astigmatism using the Alpins Method[6]; R, manifest refractive cylinder; SimK, simulated keratometry.

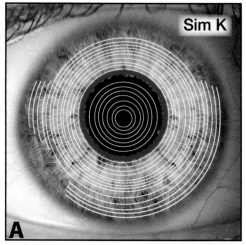

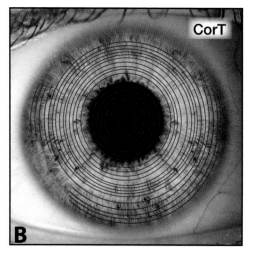

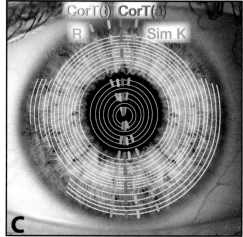

CorT also provides a consistent, standardized measure of irregular corneal astigmatism. A separate CorT calculation is made for each hemidivision of the cornea, which generates a magnitude value and a meridian value for each half of the cornea. When these calculations are added vectorially, the result is a CorT for the entire cornea. When these values are subtracted vectorially, the surgeon can determine the dioptric difference of one half of the cornea from the other half, called topographic disparity (TD), which precisely quantifies corneal irregularity and is expressed in diopters.[6,8]

The TD can be represented by the vectorial difference between the two hemidivisional CorTs on a 720° double-angle vector diagram and effectively addresses nonorthogonal and asymmetric components of irregularity in healthy astigmatic corneas[6,8] (Figure 12-3). TD allows all topographers to have a common measuring gauge for corneal irregularity.[6,9-13]

The variability of SimK values has been a point of frustration in the field, specifically regarding their meridian for the alignment of toric intraocular lenses (IOLs). I believe

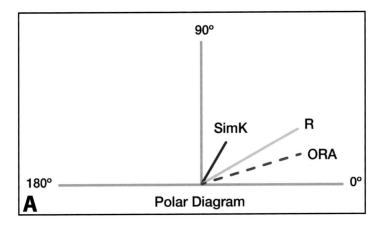

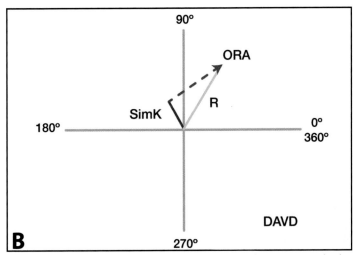

Figure 12-2. (A) The polar diagram shows SimK, the positive cylinder of the manifest refraction at the corneal plane (R), and the calculated ORA. (B) The length of the lines representing astigmatisms and vectors is based on the magnitude of the measurements and calculations. In the double-angle vector diagram (DAVD), the angles from the polar diagram have been doubled to convert to Cartesian coordinates, but the magnitude (length) of the astigmatisms and vectors remains the same. The DAVD better shows how ORA is the vectorial difference between refractive and corneal astigmatism. Since CorT has been shown superior to SimK in corresponding to both the axis and magnitude of R, it is easy to see that the ORA would be less using CorT.

that for applications where corneal astigmatism is included in the treatment plan (toric IOLs, limbal relaxing incisions with the femtosecond laser, etc), CorT will replace the SimK value, which has been the standard measure since the inception of Placido ring topography technology.[6,9,14,15] In addition to providing a measure of corneal astigmatism across the cornea as noted above, the calculated CorT of the hemidivisions of a cornea with irregular astigmatism may have future applications in treatment.[6]

Figure 12-3. This DAVD shows a planned treatment of irregular astigmatism by applying the optimal treatment separately for each corneal hemidivision, superior (TIA_{SUP}) and inferior (TIA_{INF}).[8] Two refractive astigmatism values cannot be perceived by one eye, and only summated values are shown (TIA_{NET}). Abbreviations: R, refraction; TIA, targeted induced astigmatism; T, topography.

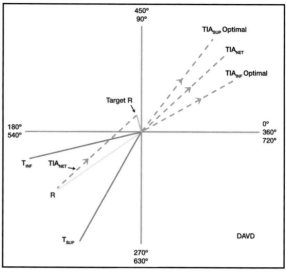

Total Corneal Power: A Deeper Dive

Since the 1990s, technological advances have allowed the measurement of corneal power with growing accuracy and detail.[6,10-12,16-18] Despite the ongoing improvements in measuring corneal power, however, no "best" or standard method has emerged to combine thousands of corneal data points into a single, possibly toric, corneal power measurement. In fact, many clinicians assume that posterior corneal astigmatism has little effect on overall refractive astigmatism, and thus, can be ignored in astigmatic calculations.[12,19]

Unfortunately, even measurements from state-of-the-art corneal tomographers seem to deviate both systematically and randomly from the manifest refractive cylinder,[11] which represents the total astigmatism of the eye including perceptual components. This situation is unlikely to be entirely resolved due to inherent differences that exist between corneal and refractive astigmatism.[10] The contribution of posterior corneal astigmatism to manifest refractive cylinder, however, is gaining the attention of investigators (Sidebar 12-1).

We have shown that CorT more accurately correlates with manifest refractive cylinder than any other common methodology for measuring the anterior corneal astigmatism—manual keratometry, SimK, corneal wavefront, etc.[6] Subsequently, we showed that a calculation we call CorT total, which includes a measure of posterior corneal astigmatism, reveals an astigmatism value for the entire cornea that is closer than the anterior CorT to manifest refractive astigmatism in magnitude and orientation.[10]

I believe that CorT total, based on total corneal astigmatism, will eventually become a standard component of surgical procedures such as toric IOL implantation, refractive "touch-ups" postkeratoplasty, limbal relaxing incisions, and topography-guided laser procedures[6,10] (Sidebar 12-2). CorT based on total corneal power can also be used for irregular corneas.[10]

Knowing the CorT total can only improve the orientation of cataract incisions, laser incisions or ablations, and toric IOL orientation required in any particular eye.

Sidebar 12-1
Posterior Corneal Astigmatism
Orientations and Magnitudes

Far from being clinically negligible, posterior corneal astigmatism has greater toricity than the anterior cornea.[20,21] Here are a few characteristics of posterior corneal astigmatism that should be kept in mind:

- Posterior corneal astigmatism optically functions like a negative lens. As a result, with-the-rule (WTR) posterior corneal astigmatism functionally adds to the total corneal against-the-rule (ATR) astigmatism.
- A number of studies[11,12,20-25] report posterior corneal astigmatism ranging from 0.26 D to 0.78 D.
- The steep posterior corneal meridian tends to be aligned closer to, but not necessarily coinciding with, the vertical 90° meridian.[11]
- With increasing age, the steep anterior corneal meridian tends to change from vertical to horizontal, while the steep posterior corneal meridian remains stable. The magnitudes of anterior and posterior corneal astigmatism are correlated when the steeper anterior meridian is aligned vertically, but not when it is aligned horizontally.[11]
- On average, corneas with anterior WTR astigmatism have about 0.5 D of WTR posterior corneal astigmatism.[11]
- Corneas with anterior ATR astigmatism have about 0.3 D of WTR posterior corneal astigmatism.[11]
- In the absence of accurate, dependable instruments to measure posterior corneal astigmatism, Koch et al[12] offered the Baylor nomogram, which can be used to adjust limbal relaxing incisions and toric intraocular lens selection based on actual anterior corneal measurements and average posterior corneal measurements found in the group's published study.

Importantly, CorT total will also provide a standardized way to compare different tomographers and the consistency of measurements across different tomographers.[6,10]

THE BENEFITS OF BEFRIENDING OCULAR RESIDUAL ASTIGMATISM

As CorT correlates with manifest refractive cylinder better than any other common clinical tool for measuring anterior corneal astigmatism,[6,10] by definition, this means that CorT is associated with lower ORA than the other methods. This is important, first, because it reveals that the other common instruments overestimate ORA. And second, lower ORA facilitates surgical planning simply by presenting surgeons with more precision and fewer cases of problematically high levels of ORA, enhancing our ability to reliably achieve excellent postoperative visual outcomes, achieving less remaining astigmatism on the cornea, and reducing the likelihood of adverse visual results.[26-31]

Sidebar 12-2
Total Corneal Astigmatism and
Ocular Residual Astigmatism

Koch et al[11] found that the amount of astigmatism contributed by the posterior cornea was being underestimated by approximately 0.22 D when the standardized keratometric index of refraction was used. Our studies[6,10] found that the mean ocular residual astigmatism (ORA) was 0.17 D lower when derived from CorT total (ORA mean = 0.53 D) than when derived from anterior CorT (ORA mean = 0.70 D). This underestimation—CorT total compared with anterior CorT—appears to be inherent when calculations include posterior corneal astigmatism.

We also found a systematic mismatch of 0.52 D between CorT total and manifest refractive cylinder. Although this difference is significantly less than for other corneal measures, it is not zero. The suggestion has been made that inclusion of posterior corneal astigmatism should account for all non-corneal astigmatism, and that the difference we are seeing is due to measurement error.[12] However, our findings support the longstanding view that manifest refractive cylinder is not caused only by corneal astigmatism, but also by noncorneal contributors such as lenticular astigmatism and processing in the visual cortex.[27,28] Additionally, refractive measurements are aligned to the center of the pupil, whereas corneal astigmatism measurements are centered on the corneal apex, which may also lead to a variable mismatch as the distance between these points vary from eye to eye.

CorT and manifest refractive cylinder can also reveal eyes with larger ORA than desirable. ORA magnitudes above 1 D may limit the acceptable outcome achievable in correcting astigmatism[29] using refractive parameters alone. For this reason, the surgeon may decide not to treat an eye or to treat spherical equivalent only. The surgeon also may opt to use the Vector Planning approach, where corneal and refractive parameters are combined to optimize and maximally reduce the resultant corneal astigmatism remaining in such cases[7,27,29,32-36] while avoiding potentially unsatisfactory outcomes.[37] The Vector Planning approach, further described in Chapter 13, has the potential for improving outcomes of astigmatism treatments for wider adoption in the future.[38] The surgeon may also counsel patients with high ORA to lower their expectations for complete correction of spherocylindrical refractive errors to more realistic levels.

CALCULATING OCULAR RESIDUAL ASTIGMATISM, CORNEAL TOPOGRAPHIC ASTIGMATISM, AND CORNEAL TOPOGRAPHIC ASTIGMATISM TOTAL: iASSORT

The calculation of ORA, CorT, and CorT total is accomplished through iAS-SORT software (ASSORT [Alpins Statistical System for Ophthalmic Refractive surgery Techniques]) (Figure 12-4), available as a standalone module interfaced with leading

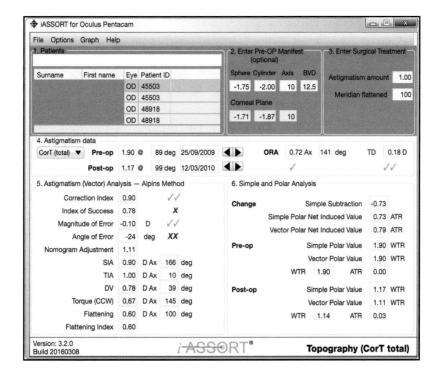

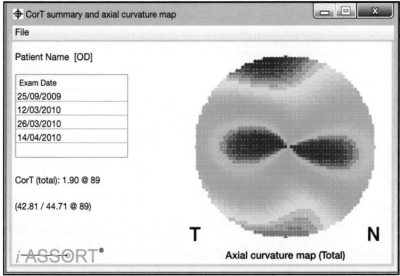

Figure 12-4. The iASSORT screen for the calculation of CorT total is shown. The program performs astigmatic analyses using the topography and/or wavefront values provided by the diagnostic instrument with which the software has been interfaced. iASSORT imports the required parameters (simulated keratometry and corneal curvature values from topography and second-order astigmatism values from aberrometry) and displays the analyses both numerically and graphically, including a reconstruction of the axial map. The Alpins Method is used to determine surgical success and refine nomograms. Other features include the calculation of topographic disparity as well as a visual indication of the success of the astigmatic treatment using symbols (ticks and crosses).

corneal topography and tomography systems (CSO Sirius [Costruzione Strumenti Oftalmici], Oculus Pentacam [Oculus], Ziemer Galilei [Ziemer], CZM Atlas [Carl Zeiss Meditec], Nidek OPD III [Nidek]).

iASSORT imports topographic data (SimK values and all corneal curvature measures captured) from topographers or second-order astigmatism values from those systems that include aberrometers. The surgeon manually enters the spherocylinder as measured by manifest refraction. From these parameters, the program calculates the ORA—the vectorial difference between the manifest refractive cylinder (or second-order spherocylinder from the wavefront aberrometry) and the corneal astigmatism (CorT or SimK). The software also calculates how much total astigmatism potentially can be corrected by reshaping the cornea.[14]

As noted above, this information can be used preoperatively to help manage patient expectations. For 25% to 30% of patients with ORA values of 1 D or more, it may not be possible to achieve the degree of astigmatism correction they might expect. Preoperative measures are also used to set a target for corneal astigmatism that minimizes total astigmatism after surgery. A target—which can be nonzero—is essential to analyze outcomes, as it provides a baseline for comparison in individuals and groups of individuals, and thus, can be used to calibrate future adjustments.[14]

A growing body of evidence supports the use of CorT and CorT total as fundamental advances in managing astigmatism in clinical studies, as well as in clinical practice. CorT better matches manifest refractive cylinder than any other measure of anterior corneal astigmatism.[6] CorT total correlates with manifest refractive cylinder better than anterior CorT.[10] Because CorT is calculated on an individual basis without the use of nomograms, it inherently outperforms corneal astigmatism measures that incorporate population-based nomogram adjustments.[10]

REFERENCES

1. Gutmark R, Guyton DL. Origins of the keratometer and its evolving role in ophthalmology. *Surv Ophthalmol.* 2010;55(5):481-497.
2. von Helmholtz H. [Uber die accommodation des auges]. *Albrecht von Graefes Archiv fur Ophthalmologie.* 1855;1:1-89.
3. Cochet P, Amiard H. [Photokeratoscopy, an element in corneal biometry]. *Bull Soc Ophtalmol Fr.* 1966;66(11):1094-1104.
4. Ludlam WM, Wittenberg S, Rosenthal J, Harris G. Photographic analysis of the ocular dioptric components. 3. The acquisition, storage, retrieval and utilization of primary data in photokeratoscopy. *Am J Optom Arch Am Acad Optom.* 1967;44(5):276-296.
5. Wilson SE, Klyce SD. Advances in the analysis of corneal topography. *Surv Ophthalmol.* 1991;35(4):269-277.
6. Alpins N, Ong JK, Stamatelatos G. New method of quantifying corneal topographic astigmatism that corresponds with manifest refractive cylinder. *J Cataract Refract Surg.* 2012;38(11):1978-1988.
7. CorT: Total Corneal Astigmatism [brochure]. ASSORT Web site. http://assort.com/ftp/ASS001%20 Cor-T%20Brochure_V2.pdf. Accessed March 23, 2015.
8. Alpins NA. Treatment of irregular astigmatism. *J Cataract Refract Surg.* 1998;24(5):634-646.
9. Ngoei E. Refractive editor's corner of the world: CorT'ing accuracy. EyeWorld Web site. http://www. eyeworld.org/article-cort-ing-accuracy. Accessed March 28, 2015.

10. Alpins NA, Ong JKY, Stamatelatos G. Corneal topographic astigmatism (CorT) to quantify total corneal astigmatism. *J Refract Surg*. 2015;31(3):182-186.

11. Koch DD, Ali SF, Weikert MP, Shirayama M, Jenkins R, Wang L. Contribution of posterior corneal astigmatism to total corneal astigmatism. *J Cataract Refract Surg*. 2012;38(12):2080-2087.

12. Koch DD, Jenkins RB, Weikert MP, Yeu E, Wang L. Correcting astigmatism with toric intraocular lenses: effect of posterior corneal astigmatism. *J Cataract Refract Surg*. 2013;39(12):1803-1809.

13. Tang M, Li Y, Avila M, Huang D. Measuring total corneal power before and after laser in situ keratomileusis with high-speed optical coherence tomography. *J Cataract Refract Surg*. 2006;32(11):1843-1850.

14. Getting more from topography. EuroTimes India Web site. http://www.eurotimesindia.org/cover-news.asp?id=262. Accessed March 23, 2015.

15. Biro A. New measurement method quantifies corneal astigmatism. Ocular Surgery News Web site. http://www.healio.com/ophthalmology/refractive-surgery/news/print/ocular-surgery-news/%7B8437E8A7-A8C3-4020-AFA6-430EC5792B3F%7D/New-measurement-method-quantifies-corneal-astigmatism. Accessed March 23, 2015.

16. Lackner B, Schmidinger G, Pieh S, Funovics MA, Skorpik C. Repeatability and reproducibility of central corneal thickness measurement with Pentacam, Orbscan, and ultrasound. *Optom Vis Sci*. 2005;82(10):892-899.

17. Wang L, Mahmoud AM, Anderson BL, Koch DD, Roberts CJ. Total corneal power estimation: ray tracing method versus gaussian optics formula. *Invest Ophthalmol Vis Sci*. 2011;52(3):1716-1722.

18. Yaylali V, Kaufman SC, Thompson HW. Corneal thickness measurements with the Orbscan Topography System and ultrasonic pachymetry. *J Cataract Refract Surg*. 1997;23(9):1345-1350.

19. Cheng LS, Tsai CY, Tsai RJ, Liou SW, Ho JD. Estimation accuracy of surgically induced astigmatism on the cornea when neglecting the posterior corneal surface measurement. *Acta Ophthalmol*. 2011;89(5):417-422.

20. Dubbelman M, Sicam VA, Van der Heijde GL. The shape of the anterior and posterior surface of the aging human cornea. *Vision Res*. 2006;46(6-7):993-1001.

21. Dunne MC, Royston JM, Barnes DA. Posterior corneal surface toricity and total corneal astigmatism. *Optom Vis Sci*. 1991;68(9):708-710.

22. Ho JD, Tsai CY, Liou SW. Accuracy of corneal astigmatism estimation by neglecting the posterior corneal surface measurement. *Am J Ophthalmol*. 2009;147(5):788-795.

23. Modis L, Jr., Langenbucher A, Seitz B. Evaluation of normal corneas using the scanning-slit topography/pachymetry system. *Cornea*. 2004;23(7):689-694.

24. Prisant O, Hoang-Xuan T, Proano C, Hernandez E, Awwad ST, Azar DT. Vector summation of anterior and posterior corneal topographical astigmatism. *J Cataract Refract Surg*. 2002;28(9):1636-1643.

25. Royston JM, Dunne MC, Barnes DA. Measurement of posterior corneal surface toricity. *Optom Vis Sci*. 1990;67(10):757-763.

26. Alio JL, Alpins N. Excimer laser correction of astigmatism: consistent terminology for better outcomes. *J Refract Surg*. 2014;30(5):294-295.

27. Alpins NA. New method of targeting vectors to treat astigmatism. *J Cataract Refract Surg*. 1997;23(1):65-75.

28. Vinas M, Sawides L, de GP, Marcos S. Perceptual adaptation to the correction of natural astigmatism. *PLoS One*. 2012;7(9):e46361.

29. Kugler L, Cohen I, Haddad W, Wang MX. Efficacy of laser in situ keratomileusis in correcting anterior and non-anterior corneal astigmatism: comparative study. *J Cataract Refract Surg*. 2010;36(10):1745-1752.

30. Qian YS, Huang J, Liu R, et al. Influence of internal optical astigmatism on the correction of myopic astigmatism by LASIK. *J Refract Surg*. 2011;27(12):863-868.

31. Frings A, Katz T, Steinberg J, Druchkiv V, Richard G, Linke SJ. Ocular residual astigmatism: effects of demographic and ocular parameters in myopic laser in situ keratomileusis. *J Cataract Refract Surg*. 2014;40(2):232-238.

32. Alpins N. Astigmatism analysis by the Alpins method. *J Cataract Refract Surg*. 2001;27(1):31-49.

33. Alpins N, Stamatelatos G. Customized photoastigmatic refractive keratectomy using combined topographic and refractive data for myopia and astigmatism in eyes with forme fruste and mild keratoconus. *J Cataract Refract Surg.* 2007;33(4):591-602.

34. Alpins N, Stamatelatos G. Clinical outcomes of laser in situ keratomileusis using combined topography and refractive wavefront treatments for myopic astigmatism. *J Cataract Refract Surg.* 2008;34(8):1250-1259.

35. Alpins N, Stamatelatos G. *Asymmetrical surgical treatment using vector planning.* In: Wang M, ed. Thorofare, NJ: SLACK Incorporated; 2008:263-268.

36. Goggin M, Alpins N, Schmid LM. Management of irregular astigmatism. *Curr Opin Ophthalmol.* 2000;11(4):260-266.

37. Solomon KD, Fernandez de Castro LE, Sandoval HP, et al. LASIK world literature review: quality of life and patient satisfaction. *Ophthalmology.* 2009;116(4):691-701.

38. Kugler LJ, Wang M. Corneal topography: what will the upcoming decade bring? In: Wang M, editor. *Corneal Topography: A Guide for Clinical Application in the Wavefront Er*a. Thorofare, NJ: SLACK Incorporated; 2012:259-262.

Chapter 13

Vector Planning Approach
Optimizing Both Corneal and Refractive Astigmatism

THE FEAT OF KEEPING UP

I told my doctor I broke my leg in two places. He told me to quit going to those places.
—Henny Youngman

In both cataract and refractive surgery, there is a long tradition of careful and customized planning. Perhaps, no specialist pays more attention to planning than the ophthalmologist, as the outcome of these interventions is largely based on a most subjective assessment—the postoperative vision as experienced by the individual patient. These are procedures with small margins of error, possessing outcomes to which patients can devote intensive scrutiny both immediately after surgery and for the remainder of their lives. Although some patients are more critical than others, all patients know what they see.

I believe that ophthalmologists are generally conservative by nature. Yet, we have performed an amazing feat. To provide the best care to patients, our instinct is to plan, plan, and then plan some more. Over the years, we have managed to accomplish this conservative, responsible planning in the face of mind-boggling and often rapid advances. To do the best for our patients, we had to keep up with advances and adjust our practices accordingly. For example, at one point in the past, the implantation of an intraocular lens (IOL) after cataract extraction was considered in some quarters to be tantamount to malpractice. Later on, not that long after, the opposite could be said if an IOL were not offered to a cataract patient. Ophthalmologists of the time were well-advised to consider this development in their surgical plans.

Since the last cryogenic intracapsular cataract extraction was performed as a routine procedure in the developed world, there have probably been thousands of advances in cataract and refractive surgery that required a change in the surgical plan. Some of these were fundamental and huge; some were incremental and small. Any ophthalmologist in clinical practice for a while has incorporated important changes, keeping pace with the literature, pursuing continuing medical education, attending professional conferences, and listening to the great teachers in our field, who will be the first to admit that they are also students. We are all students, and will continue to be students for as long as we practice. For the benefit of our patients, we must continue our amazing feat.

Alpins N. *Practical Astigmatism:*
Planning and Analysis (pp 105-112).
© 2018 SLACK Incorporated.

In my view, the modern corneal and refractive surgeon would be well-advised to incorporate measurements of both corneal and refractive astigmatism in the surgical plan—not simply to take these measurements, but to submit them to what I call the Vector Planning approach. Like Henny Youngman's leg broken in two places, ophthalmologists will not go to those places by considering either corneal or refractive astigmatism alone. Instead, ophthalmologists will use both astigmatism domains to develop an optimal plan for the individual patient, continuing our tradition of careful, customized planning.

Advances in Measurement

Measurements of both refractive and corneal astigmatism are key ingredients of the Vector Planning approach specifically, and of the Alpins Method in general. As in ophthalmology and almost any other field, where there are measurements, there is technology. The traditional measurement of manifest refraction has been joined by wavefront analysis[1-4]; the measurement of corneal astigmatism, once the province of keratometry alone, was supplemented first by corneal topography (anterior corneal astigmatism), and more recently, by corneal tomography (total corneal astigmatism).[5-11]

Wavefront analysis adds a measure of higher-order aberrations—such as spherical aberration, coma, and foils—to the lower-order aberrations of myopia, hyperopia, and astigmatism revealed by traditional refraction.[1] However, a refractive procedure based solely on wavefront analysis is little different from a refractive procedure based solely on traditional manifest refraction. Either way, corneal astigmatism is ignored at the potential cost of less desirable results.[1,12-18] Combining wavefront with topography using a Vector Planning approach has shown better outcomes than using wavefront alone.[1,14-16,19]

Corneal tomography provides a measure of total corneal power. The technology, which I believe one day will be widely available and routinely used, is a valuable complement to corneal topography,[5-11] providing an objective measure that is closer than topography to the subjective measure of manifest refraction. Closer, but not identical—total corneal power often differs in orientation or magnitude from astigmatism measured by refraction.[8-11]

This difference between corneal and refractive astigmatism, no matter how refined the technology becomes in measuring either domain, is inherent, and will likely continue to be unavoidable. Thus, ocular residual astigmatism (ORA), defined as the vectorial difference between corneal and refractive astigmatism expressed in diopters and degrees,[14,16,20,21] will persist as a common finding in smaller or larger amounts.

As described in Chapter 9, ORA is the absolute minimum amount of astigmatism that will remain in the eye after refractive surgery. It is the amount of corneal astigmatism that will remain (a nonzero target) if only refractive astigmatism is corrected, and the amount of refractive astigmatism that will remain (again, a nonzero target) if only corneal astigmatism is corrected.

The best theoretical outcome or the maximum possible reduction in astigmatism occurs when the remaining astigmatism is equivalent to the ORA.[21] The remaining astigmatism can be refractive, corneal, or any combination of both. Using the Vector Planning approach, the surgeon can choose the proportion of any of the ORA to remain in the theoretical refraction, while reducing the targeted corneal astigmatism.[22]

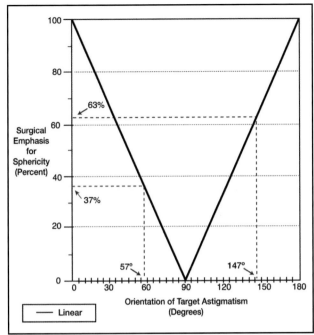

Figure 13-1. ASSORT calculates "optimal treatment" based on the linear relationship shown here. Future research may determine that the actual relationship is nonlinear or otherwise varies from the graph shown. In this example, the meridian of target topography is 147°, which lies 57° from a with-the-rule orientation of 90°. Using this linear relationship, the surgeon may decide to apportion 57° of 90° (63.3%) emphasis to a topography-based goal of zero astigmatism (147° intersects the linear emphasis line at 63%). This results in a 63% emphasis on the correction of refractive astigmatism and 37% on correcting corneal astigmatism. (Reprinted from *Journal of Cataract & Refractive Surgery*, 23/1, Alpins NA, New method of targeting vectors to treat astigmatism, 11, Copyright 1997, with permission from Elsevier.)

THE VECTOR PLANNING APPROACH: A MATTER OF EMPHASIS

The Vector Planning approach allows surgeons to customize astigmatic treatment emphasis based on the following principles[21-24]:

- Less corneal astigmatism remaining is preferable to more (about 7% of patients preoperatively have an ORA that could result in an increased corneal astigmatism if treatment is based exclusively on refractive cylinder[21]).
- When remaining astigmatism is unavoidable after correction, then a with-the-rule orientation for distance vision is more favorable than an against-the-rule orientation.

The guiding principle of the Vector Planning approach is this: to favor a goal of corneal sphericity when the astigmatism being targeted is in a less than favorable orientation, such as oblique or against the rule.[20] The Vector Planning approach allows a customized approach, optimizing treatment according to a patient's existing corneal and optical parameters.[22] Less overall corneal astigmatism is targeted by orienting the maximum ablation closer to the principal corneal meridian. Importantly, the establishment of targets allows valid postoperative analysis of astigmatic results, both corneal and refractive.[20-22]

The ASSORT (Alpins Statistical System for Ophthalmic Refractive surgery Techniques) program includes an "optimal treatment" feature that calculates laser treatment parameters to correct the maximum amount of astigmatism (ORA) while leaving the least possible corneal astigmatism at the unfavorable, against-the-rule orientation[21] (Figure 13-1). This could be considered a type of "automated" Vector Planning approach

Figure 13-2. ASSORT can generate tables such as the ones shown here. (A) Surgical emphasis can be calculated to correct 100% of refractive astigmatism, (B) 100% of corneal astigmatism, (C) or any midpoint between the 2.

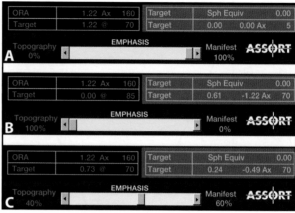

as opposed to the "manual" Vector Planning approach described below. The surgeon, of course, decides whether to use either or neither approach.

Optimal treatment calculates laser settings that put a greater emphasis on the reduction of refractive cylinder the closer the remaining corneal astigmatism is to 90° (with-the-rule). In one paradigm that can be employed if the meridian of target topography is 90°, 100% of the treatment emphasis will be devoted to the correction of refractive astigmatism. If the meridian of target topography is 180°, 100% of the treatment emphasis will be devoted to correcting the topographic astigmatism. Optimal treatment seeks to achieve less corneal astigmatism than if treating by refraction alone, with an attempt to influence its orientation favorably.[25-27]

The ASSORT program can generate excimer laser treatment parameters using the Vector Planning approach (with emphasis bars); examples of various treatment paradigms are shown in Figure 13-2. The double-angle vector diagrams (DAVDs) in Figure 13-3 are graphical examples of the concept shown in Figure 13-2.

100% Correction of Refractive Astigmatism

A 100% emphasis on correcting refractive astigmatism leaves the topographic target at a level equivalent to the ORA, but at 90° to the ORA to neutralize the internal astigmatism; in this case, +0.46 D at an axis of 98° (Figure 13-2A).

100% Correction of Corneal Astigmatism

A 100% emphasis on corneal astigmatism will result in a spherical cornea (Figure 13-2B). The refractive target, however, will be sphere +0.23 D, cylinder −0.46 D, at axis 98°, always targeting a spherical equivalent of zero.

A Divided Emphasis

An emphasis split between corneal astigmatism (41%) and refractive astigmatism (59%) represents a surgical balance of the two targeted zero-astigmatism goals. The topographic target is +0.27 D at 98° and the refractive target is sphere +0.10 D, cylinder −0.19 D at axis 98° (Figure 13-2C). This results in a non-zero target for both corneal and

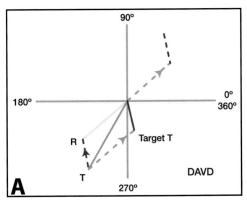

Figure 13-3. (A) DAVDs (with corresponding emphasis bars, lower left) show refractive (R) and topographic (T) astigmatism vectors, with planned treatments aimed at correcting 100% of refractive astigmatism, (B) 100% of corneal astigmatism, and (C) a 50-50 midpoint treatment.

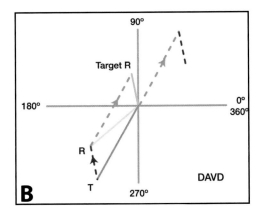

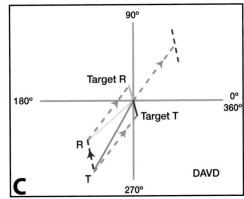

refractive astigmatism. It is important to note that with the Vector Planning approach, there is always a targeted spherical equivalent of zero in the postoperative refraction – where the patient is spectacle free and least likely to notice any reduction in their vision.

IRREGULAR ASTIGMATISM: VECTOR PLANNING APPROACH × 2

As many as 40% of "normal" corneas with a toric refractive error can be said to have primary irregular astigmatism.[28] Irregularity may exist across the corneal hemidivision as a difference in dioptric magnitude (asymmetry) or orientation (nonorthogonal) or both. I have described topographic disparity (TD) as a tool for quantifying corneal irregularity.[29] TD is the dioptric separation between the two corneal hemidivisions as shown on a 720° DAVD, described in greater detail in Chapter 16. Irregularity is said to be significant in eyes with a TD > 1.00 D, which is found in 44% of eyes with treatable astigmatism.[28,29]

The Vector Planning approach can be applied to formulate separate surgical plans and unique targeted induced astigmatism vector values for each hemidivision. Inevitably, excimer lasers will be able to deliver the separate hemidivisional treatment required. The goal will be what I call reduction and regularization, which is described in Chapter 17. The reward will be better visual acuity and enhanced overall visual performance.

Sidebar 13-1
ORA and Vector Planning in Practice

Vector Planning should be used in cases where a discrepancy exists between corneal and refractive astigmatism. This discrepancy is quantified through a calculation called ORA. So how much ORA can be expected in a typical patient population? And how much ORA makes Vector Planning clinically relevant?

In consecutive patients receiving photorefractive surgery, ORA ranged from 0.73 D to 0.81 D[14,18,20] and exceeded 1.00 D in 34% of eyes.[20] In a study introducing the concept of corneal topographic astigmatism (CorT) total, based on total corneal power using measures from multiple Placido rings (see Chapter 12), we found a mean ORA magnitude of 0.53 D with a 0.30-D standard deviation.[9] Interestingly, the study also found a systematic mismatch of 0.52 D between CorT total and manifest refractive cylinder. This finding supports the longstanding view that manifest refractive cylinder is not caused only by corneal astigmatism, anterior and posterior, but also by noncorneal contributors such as lenticular astigmatism and processing in the visual cortex.[21,35]

Any decision to adjust laser settings using Vector Planning is the surgeon's. Excessive target corneal astigmatism (more than 0.75 D) can be avoided by an increased treatment emphasis on topographic correction (Figure 13-2). For patients with an ORA > 1.25 D, I tend to "share the load" between the cornea and refraction by using a 50-50 emphasis (Figure 13-3) or by using proportionate or target meridian paradigms. Surgeons can calculate the laser settings by employing the published mathematics[20-22]; however, the settings are more easily generated by the ASSORT program, which can target corneal astigmatism at any meridian the surgeon chooses when using customized mode.

THE ULTIMATE APPLICATION OF THE ALPINS METHOD

In recent years, the importance of the Alpins Method in studying and reporting the results of refractive surgery has become apparent.[30-34] Researchers finally have a useful, comprehensive, common language in their approach to astigmatism, but in terms of the sheer number of people affected, the Vector Planning approach may be the method's most significant application. Using the Vector Planning approach, every refractive surgeon can offer some level of improved care to every patient.

Better vision, of course, is the most desirable outcome. But the Vector Planning approach also offers critical help in cultivating more realistic patient expectations, offering alternative procedures, or even avoiding surgical intervention altogether. These attributes also contribute to increased quality of care.

REFERENCES

1. Alpins NA, Schmid L. Combining vector planning with wavefront analysis to optimize laser in-situ keratomileusis outcomes. In: Krueger RR, Applegate RA, MacRae SM, eds. *Wavefront Customized Visual Correction: The Quest for Super Vision II.* Thorofare, New Jersey: SLACK Incorporated; 2004:317-328.

2. Carones F, Vigo L, Scandola E, Sorace SG. Expanded range customcornea algorithms for myopia and astigmatism: one-month results. *J Refract Surg.* 2004;20(5):S619-S623.

3. Mastropasqua L, Nubile M, Ciancaglini M, Toto L, Ballone E. Prospective randomized comparison of wavefront-guided and conventional photorefractive keratectomy for myopia with the meditec MEL 70 laser. *J Refract Surg.* 2004;20(5):422-431.

4. Winkler von MC, Huber A, Gabler B et al. Wavefront-guided laser epithelial keratomileusis with the wavelight concept system 500. *J Refract Surg.* 2004;20(5):S565-S569.

5. Lackner B, Schmidinger G, Pieh S, Funovics MA, Skorpik C. Repeatability and reproducibility of central corneal thickness measurement with Pentacam, Orbscan, and ultrasound. *Optom Vis Sci.* 2005;82(10):892-899.

6. Wang L, Mahmoud AM, Anderson BL, Koch DD, Roberts CJ. Total corneal power estimation: ray tracing method versus gaussian optics formula. *Invest Ophthalmol Vis Sci.* 2011;52(3):1716-1722.

7. Yaylali V, Kaufman SC, Thompson HW. Corneal thickness measurements with the Orbscan Topography System and ultrasonic pachymetry. *J Cataract Refract Surg.* 1997;23(9):1345-1350.

8. Alpins N, Ong JK, Stamatelatos G. New method of quantifying corneal topographic astigmatism that corresponds with manifest refractive cylinder. *J Cataract Refract Surg.* 2012;38(11):1978-1988.

9. Alpins NA, Ong JKY, Stamatelatos G. Corneal topographic astigmatism (CorT) to quantify total corneal astigmatism. *J Refract Surg.* 2015;31(3):182-186.

10. Koch DD, Ali SF, Weikert MP, Shirayama M, Jenkins R, Wang L. Contribution of posterior corneal astigmatism to total corneal astigmatism. *J Cataract Refract Surg.* 2012;38(12):2080-2087.

11. Koch DD, Jenkins RB, Weikert MP, Yeu E, Wang L. Correcting astigmatism with toric intraocular lenses: effect of posterior corneal astigmatism. *J Cataract Refract Surg.* 2013;39(12):1803-1809.

12. Alpins NA. Wavefront technology: a new advance that fails to answer old questions on corneal vs. refractive astigmatism correction. *J Refract Surg.* 2002;18(6):737-739.

13. Walsh MJ. Is the future of refractive surgery based on corneal topography or wavefront? Ocular Surgery News Web site. http://www.healio.com/ophthalmology/refractive-surgery/news/print/ocular-surgery-news/%7Bdf8c4698-b178-47f7-83cb-b3c890916b7f%7D/is-the-future-of-refractive-surgery-based-on-corneal-topography-or-wavefront. Published August 1, 2000. Accessed August 9, 2014.

14. Alpins N, Stamatelatos G. Customized photoastigmatic refractive keratectomy using combined topographic and refractive data for myopia and astigmatism in eyes with forme fruste and mild keratoconus. *J Cataract Refract Surg.* 2007;33(4):591-602.

15. Alpins N, Stamatelatos G. Clinical outcomes of laser in situ keratomileusis using combined topography and refractive wavefront treatments for myopic astigmatism. *J Cataract Refract Surg.* 2008;34(8):1250-1259.

16. Alpins NA, Stamatelatos G. Combined wavefront and topography approach to refractive surgery treatments. In: Wang M, ed. *Corneal Topography in the Wavefront Era: A Guide for Clinical Application.* Thorofare, NJ: SLACK Incorporated; 2006:139-143.

17. Kugler L, Cohen I, Haddad W, Wang MX. Efficacy of laser in situ keratomileusis in correcting anterior and non-anterior corneal astigmatism: comparative study. *J Cataract Refract Surg.* 2010;36(10):1745-1752.

18. Qian YS, Huang J, Liu R, et al. Influence of internal optical astigmatism on the correction of myopic astigmatism by LASIK. *J Refract Surg.* 2011;27(12):863-868.

19. Alpins N. Combining wavefront and topography data [letter]. *J Cataract Refract Surg.* 2005;31(4):646-647.

20. Alpins N. Astigmatism analysis by the Alpins method. *J Cataract Refract Surg.* 2001;27(1):31-49.

21. Alpins NA. New method of targeting vectors to treat astigmatism. *J Cataract Refract Surg.* 1997;23(1):65-75.

22. Alpins NA. A new method of analyzing vectors for changes in astigmatism. *J Cataract Refract Surg.* 1993;19(4):524-533.

23. Alpins NA, Terry CM. Astigmatism: LASIK, LASEK, and PRK. In: Roy FH, Arzabe CW, eds. *Master Techniques in Cataract and Refractive Surgery.* Thorofare, NJ: SLACK Incorporated; 2004:151-160.

24. Mimouni M, Nemet A, Pokroy R, Sela T, Munzer G, Kaiserman I. The effect of astigmatism axis on visual acuity. *Eur J Ophthalmol.* 27(3):308-311.

25. Eggers H. Estimation of uncorrected visual acuity in malingerers. *Arch Ophthalmol.* 1945;33:23-27.

26. Friedman B. Acceptance of weak cylinders at paradoxic axes. *Arch Ophthalmol.* 1940;23:720-726.

27. Sawusch MR, Guyton DL. Optimal astigmatism to enhance depth of focus after cataract surgery. *Ophthalmology.* 1991;98:1025-1029.

28. Goggin M, Alpins N, Schmid LM. Management of irregular astigmatism. *Curr Opin Ophthalmol.* 2000;11(4):260-266.

29. Alpins NA. Treatment of irregular astigmatism. *J Cataract Refract Surg.* 1998;24(5):634-646.

30. Author Information Pack. American Academy of Ophthalmology Web site. https://www.elsevier.com/wps/find/journaldescription.cws_home/620418?generatepdf=true. Accessed January 19, 2016.

31. Information for Authors. American Society of Cataract and Refractive Surgery Web site. http://www.jcrsjournal.org/content/authorinfo#info. Accessed September 1, 2016.

32. Reinstein DZ, Archer TJ, Randleman JB. JRS standard for reporting astigmatism outcomes of refractive surgery [editorial]. *J Refract Surg.* 2014;30(10):654-659.

33. Reinstein DZ, Archer TJ, Srinivasan S, Mamalis N, Kohnen T, Dupps Jr WJ, Randleman JB. Standard for reporting refractive outcomes of intraocular lens-based refractive surgery. Journal Cataract Refract Surg. 2017;43(4);435-439.

34. Reinstein DZ, Randleman JB, Archer TJ, et al. JRS standard for reporting outcomes of intraocular lens based refractive surgery. *J Refract Surg.* 2017;33(4):218-222.

35. Vinas M, Sawides L, de GP, Marcos S. Perceptual adaptation to the correction of natural astigmatism. *PLoS One.* 2012;7(9):e46361.

Chapter 14

Corneal Astigmatism
Less Is More

MILLIONS OF YEARS IN THE MAKING

Here's where it gets magical: The Alpins Method allows the practitioner to clearly understand that "less is more" and then deliberately chart a course clinically to obtain more for less.

Let me explain.

As discussed in Chapter 9 and elsewhere herein, the Alpins Method is used to calculate a value called ocular residual astigmatism (ORA)[1-4], which is the vectorial difference—expressed in diopters and degrees—between refractive and corneal astigmatism. ORA is the irreducible, inescapable, minimum amount of astigmatism that can remain in the eye after refractive surgery. The ORA can be insignificant (for people whose refractive and corneal astigmatism are of identical or nearly identical magnitude and orientation) or substantial (for people whose refractive and corneal astigmatism differ by about 1 D or greater and/or demonstrate a significant difference in orientation). Using the Alpins Method, the surgeon can choose to target 100% of laser treatment on refractive astigmatism, 100% on corneal astigmatism, or any combination of refractive and corneal astigmatism totaling 100%, which ideally maintains the ORA—the minimum amount of astigmatism in the visual system (Figure 14-1).

We have discussed how a refractive surgical procedure based solely on refraction—including refraction from wavefront analysis—ignores corneal astigmatism at the potential cost of less desirable results.[2,4-10] We also believe that corneal tomography, and its measure of total corneal power, is a valuable tool,[11-17] providing a metric that is closer than anterior topography to the subjective measure of manifest refraction (see Chapter 12). Total corneal power, however, often differs in orientation or magnitude from astigmatism measured by refraction.[14-17] This difference between corneal and refractive astigmatism, no matter how refined the technology used to measure either domain, is inherent and unavoidable. Nature herself promises us that ORA will persist as a common finding no matter how accurate our measurement tools.

Alpins N. *Practical Astigmatism:
Planning and Analysis* (pp 113-122).
© 2018 SLACK Incorporated.

Figure 14-1. Emphasis bars generated by the ASSORT program calculate treatment settings along the full spectrum of treatment possibilities, where remaining astigmatism in the ocular system is at an absolute minimum (the vector of ORA). (A) The surgeon can choose to target 100% of laser treatment on refractive astigmatism, (B) 100% on corneal astigmatism, (C) or split the difference between refractive and corneal astigmatism—in this case, a 59% emphasis on refraction and a 41% emphasis on topography. (Reprinted with permission from Alpins NA, Terry CM. Astigmatism: LASIK, LASEK, and PRK. In: Roy FH, Arzabe CW, eds. *Master Techniques in Cataract and Refractive Surgery.* Thorofare, NJ: SLACK Incorporated; 2004:151-160.)

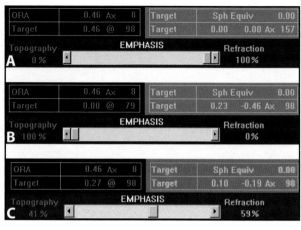

We know that the Vector Planning approach (Chapter 13) combined with wavefront treatment parameters provides better outcomes than using wavefront parameters alone.[4,8,18] It is through the Vector Planning approach that we can discern the "less-is-more" phenomenon. Although not quite magical, the phenomenon appears to leverage a natural flexibility baked into human vision over the course of our evolution (Sidebar 14-1).

LESS ON REFRACTION, MORE ON CORNEA

In clinical practice, for the many patients having significant ORA, we find that placing less emphasis on the correction of refractive cylinder (and more on the correction of corneal astigmatism) results in better postoperative manifest refractive cylinder than predicted (Figure 14-4). Quite simply, here is the point: Less is more. By apportioning some of the treatment emphasis to correcting the corneal astigmatism, the patient often enjoys better visual results than might be expected. The practitioner can vary the emphasis depending on various factors, as described in greater detail below.

Keep in mind that the best theoretical outcome or the maximum possible reduction in astigmatism occurs when the remaining astigmatism is equivalent to the ORA.[3] The remaining astigmatism can be refractive, topographic, or any combination of both. Using the Vector Planning approach, the surgeon chooses the proportion of any of the ORA remaining in the theoretical refraction, while reducing the targeted corneal astigmatism.[19] In our experience, a 60:40 ratio—with 60% of the emphasis on refraction and 40% of the emphasis on the cornea—is the "sweet spot" in optimizing visual results, as shown in Figure 14-5.

Using ASSORT (Alpins Statistical System for Ophthalmic Refractive surgery Techniques; Figure 14-5), the practitioner enters the patient's corneal and refractive measurements based on the results of the clinical examination. Values such as ORA,

Sidebar 14-1
How the Eye Impressed Charles Darwin

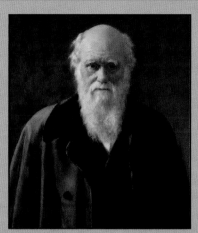

Figure 14-2. Portrait of Charles Darwin (1809-1882), the scientist and author of *On the Origin of Species*.[32] (Reprinted with permission from National Portrait Gallery, http://www.npg.org.uk/collections/search/use-this-image.php?mkey=mw01728.)

The complexity of the eye led Charles Darwin (Figure 14-2) to pen a paragraph[30] that is still widely taken out of context to support creationism.[31] Here's the passage from *The Origin of Species*:

To suppose that the eye with all its inimitable contrivances for adjusting the focus to different distances, for admitting different amounts of light, and for the correction of spherical and chromatic aberration, could have been formed by natural selection, seems, I freely confess, absurd in the highest degree. Yet reason tells me, that if numerous gradations from a simple and imperfect eye to one complex and perfect can be shown to exist, each grade being useful to its possessor, as is certainly the case; if further, the eye ever varies and the variations be inherited, as is likewise certainly the case and if such variations should be useful to any animal under changing conditions of life, then the difficulty of believing that a perfect and complex eye could be formed by natural selection, though insuperable by our imagination, should not be considered as subversive of the theory.

Creationists, as one might expect, freely quote the first sentence of the passage.

Unlike bones, whose evolutionary development is clear in the fossil record, soft tissues rarely fossilize, and when they do, little structural detail can be worked out. Relatively recent studies have compared embryos, eye structure, and genes across species to pinpoint when key traits arose. Results suggest that our type of eye—common across vertebrates—developed over the course of less than 100 million years, evolving from a simple light sensor[33] (Figure 14-3) around 600 million years ago to an optically and neurologically sophisticated organ by 500 million years ago.[34]

(continued)

axes, targets, corneal/spectacle plane adjustments, etc, are calculated automatically based on routine refractive surgical analytics, as well as the published mathematics inherent to the Alpins Method.[1-4,7,8,14,15,19-29] Adjustments for variations between lasers can also be applied. In addition to the calculations needed to generate the values in the tables, polar vector graphs are created, as shown. The corneal topographic astigmatism (CorT) is calculated[14,15] using the iASSORT program. Shifting the emphasis bar from 100% refraction (manifest) to 100% topography (CorT) provides the surgeon with a valuable

Sidebar 14-1 (continued)
How the Eye Impressed Charles Darwin

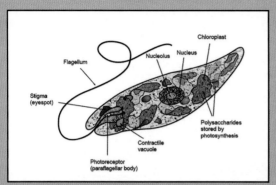

Figure 14-3. The "eyespot" of unicellular organisms such as the euglena, shown here, is likely the earliest predecessor of the human eye. Called a stigma in the euglena, the eyespot senses ambient light, but cannot distinguish shapes or the direction of the light source. Located at its anterior end, the euglena's stigma is a small patch of red pigment over light-sensitive crystals. Together with the leading flagellum, the eyespot allows the euglena to move, usually toward the light to assist in photosynthesis.[33]

"Pessimistic" calculations have shown that the vertebrate eye could have evolved from a patch of photoreceptors in less than 364,000 years. The calculations overestimate the time required between key evolutionary stages and assume that a generation is one year, which is common in small animals.[33,35]

According to Trevor Lamb, a vision scientist at the John Curtin School of Medical Research and the Australian National University in Canberra:

The latest evolutionary findings on the human eye "put the nail in the coffin of irreducible complexity and beautifully support Darwin's idea. They also explain why the eye, far from being a perfectly engineered piece of machinery, exhibits a number of major flaws—these flaws are the scars of evolution. Natural selection does not, as some might think, result in perfection. It tinkers with the material available to it, sometimes to odd effect."[34]

perspective of that particular patient's situation. As with the box score in American baseball, which provides an overall sense of the game to one who understands how to read it, after a little practice, the screen grab shown in Figure 14-5 affords the surgeon an overall sense of the case.

Any significant ORA ought to catch our attention. A scroll of the emphasis bar will show a target induced astigmatism vector (TIA) that moves from superimposition on one domain (for example, manifest refraction) to superimposition on the other (topography, or CorT). An intermediate emphasis (for example, 60% refraction and 40% topography) will display the TIA between the two, together with the magnitude (diopters) and orientation (degrees) of the vector.

For preoperative values, we now routinely use patients' CorT[14,15] and manifest refractions. Topography values can also be taken from any corneal measuring device (IOLMaster [Zeiss], Lenstar [Haag-Streit], etc). CorT,[14,15] described in greater detail in

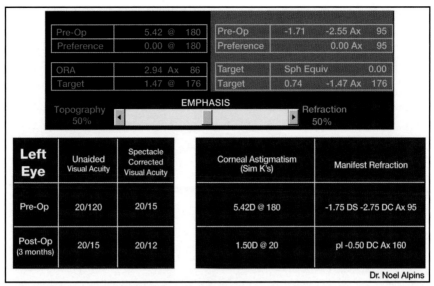

Pre-Op	5.42 @ 180	Pre-Op	-1.71	-2.55 Ax 95
Preference	0.00 @ 180	Preference		0.00 Ax 95
ORA	2.94 Ax 86	Target	Sph Equiv	0.00
Target	1.47 @ 176	Target	0.74	-1.47 Ax 176

EMPHASIS

Topography 50% — Refraction 50%

Left Eye	Unaided Visual Acuity	Spectacle Corrected Visual Acuity	Corneal Astigmatism (Sim K's)	Manifest Refraction
Pre-Op	20/120	20/15	5.42D @ 180	-1.75 DS -2.75 DC Ax 95
Post-Op (3 months)	20/15	20/12	1.50D @ 20	pl -0.50 DC Ax 160

Dr. Noel Alpins

Figure 14-4. A patient with keratoconus[2] has ORA of 2.94 D axis 86°. The surgeon chooses a treatment emphasis of 50% refractive and 50% corneal astigmatism. The target refractive cylinder is thus 1.47 D, with a spherical equivalent of zero, and the target corneal astigmatism is likewise 1.47 D. After surgery, the measured corneal astigmatism is 1.50 D, but the refractive cylinder is 0.50 D—much lower than theoretically expected (note that the target spherical equivalent is zero). We believe this "less-is-more" effect is due to the reduced corneal astigmatism resulting from the 50:50 treatment emphasis. In this case, treatment based on refraction alone would have left all of the ORA (2.94 D) on the cornea.

Chapter 12, correlates with manifest refractive cylinder more closely than does simulated keratometry (SimK) for reasons that include a more extensive capture of data across the cornea. SimK is based on corneal astigmatism in the 3-mm zone. In contrast, CorT is based on data across a wide annular region of the cornea, gathered from all complete Placido rings. Since CorT does a better job in approaching the magnitude and axis of manifest refractive cylinder than the other commonly used measures of corneal astigmatism, the calculated ORA usually is less using CorT than it would be with other commonly used methods.[36]

EMPHASIS AS DISPLAYED IN DOUBLE-ANGLE VECTOR DIAGRAMS

Double-angle vector diagrams (DAVDs) have been used in many other chapters. I show them again in Figure 14-6 to supplement the concept of treatment emphasis. DAVDs have limited utility in clinical situations, but are fundamental to the calculations used in the Alpins Method. You might think of DAVDs as operating "behind the scenes" in performing these calculations; obviously, most clinicians think of astigmatic refractive correction in terms of the polar coordinates, as graphed in Figure 14-5.

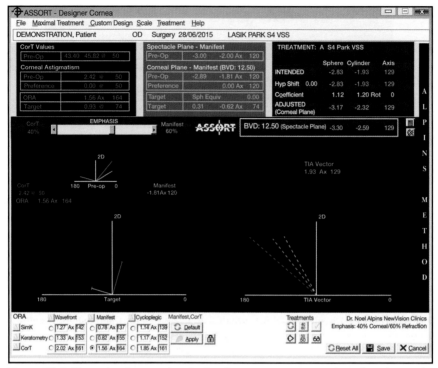

Figure 14-5. The patient's corneal and refractive measurements are based on the results of the clinical examination; other values are calculated automatically (image based on screen grab from the ASSORT program). The CorT value[14,15] is calculated using the iASSORT program. Polar vector graphs are created, as shown. Shifting the emphasis bar from 100% refraction (manifest) to 100% topography (CorT) provides the surgeon with the range of possible treatment settings and a graphical representation of the TIA throughout the range.

CLINICAL LESSONS LEARNED

As with the practice of medicine in general, incorporating astigmatism correction into refractive and cataract surgical practice is nine parts science and one part art. There are general areas of agreement as well as areas where disagreement is common among those of us who practice and teach refractive and cataract surgery. For example, many ophthalmologists might contend that there is more than "one part art" in ophthalmology. But perhaps that debate should be left for another time (one thing is certain—it's not difficult to find areas of debate in ophthalmology).

Refractive surgeons target patients to have zero postoperative astigmatism—neither with-the-rule (WTR) nor against-the-rule (ATR).[37] Although each patient's unique situation must be considered, in general, I tend to believe that a small amount of WTR astigmatism—0.25 D to 0.75 D—is a reasonable goal, especially in light of a long-term ATR shift that occurs with aging.[38]

A number of "rules of thumb" have become apparent to me over the course of my clinical practice (Sidebar 14-2). More controlled studies are planned or under way, of course, which will help to formalize these concepts. I offer these observations, though, in the event that they might prove helpful.

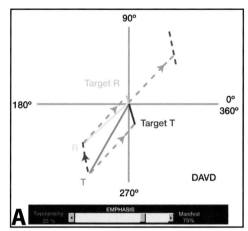
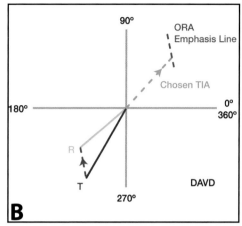

Figure 14-6. (A) DAVDs help demonstrate how the Cartesian vector calculations are performed. The relative lengths of the refraction vector (R) and topographic vector (T) reflect the R and T measurements in diopters; their relative axes are doubled from the orientations actually measured. The practitioner decides on a 25:75 treatment emphasis—that is, 25% of the ORA will remain in the refractive cylinder, and 75% of the ORA will remain on the cornea postoperatively. (B) The target corneal astigmatism (Target T) and target refractive astigmatism (Target R) are shown. Any selected emphasis comprises the target induced astigmatism vector (Chosen TIA) with treatment resulting in the minimal possible astigmatism, represented by the emphasis line of the ocular residual astigmatism (ORA Emphasis Line). The selected 25:75 treatment emphasis is shown.

Sidebar 14-2
"Rules of Thumb" for Determining Treatment Emphasis

Here are a number of concepts to consider when deciding on treatment emphasis using Vector Planning for a refractive surgery patient with astigmatism:

1. Selecting "optimal treatment,"[3] which is built into the ASSORT program, where the emphasis is determined using a linear or cosine relationship to the targeted astigmatism orientation (see Chapter 6).
2. Using average emphasis from previous treatments (40% topography, 60% refraction).
3. Leaving no more than 0.75 D on the cornea and/or <0.50 D in the refraction in cases where the ORA ≤ 1.25 D.
4. Splitting the ORA at the midpoint using a 50-50 emphasis (50% topography, 50% refraction).
5. Choosing a treatment emphasis that is proportional to the preoperative corneal and refractive astigmatism—that is, a treatment emphasis that maintains the same ratio between corneal and refractive astigmatism as exists preoperatively.
6. Selecting the minimum astigmatic treatment (or target induced astigmatism) based on the parabolic curve that exists between the extremes of topographic and refractive treatments.

The 60:40 (refraction-to-topography) apportionment of treatment emphasis appears to hold true for patients with ORA values up to 1.25 D. Applying 40% less of the ORA to the cornea in these cases seems reasonable. With ORA > 1.25 D, as we may see in patients with keratoconus,[2] a 50:50 emphasis may be preferred; that is, an increased emphasis of corneal astigmatism reduction vs the 60:40 emphasis.

WTR vs ATR astigmatic target corneal orientation is also a consideration. I see ATR astigmatism as less favorable, as many of the cues in the world around us have a vertical orientation favoring the visual perception of those who have WTR astigmatism. For patients with ATR target corneal astigmatism, I tend to go more to the left on the emphasis bar (in the ASSORT treatment screen), thus, leaving less astigmatism on the cornea. The opposite is true for patients with WTR target corneal astigmatism; that is, I tend to go more to the right on the emphasis bar, leaving the more favorable astigmatism on the cornea and less in the refraction.

Finally, as included in the accompanying rules of thumb (and shown in Figure 14-5), sliding the treatment emphasis from 100% refraction to 100% cornea generates a TIA line on the polar diagram that swings from superimposition on the vector to correct refractive cylinder, to superimposition on the vector for corneal astigmatism, by definition. However, especially in patients with higher levels of ORA, the length of the TIA can be seen to shorten in the intermediate zone between 100% refraction and 100% cornea. That is because the magnitude (hence the length) of the TIA follows a parabolic curve between the two extremes in treatment emphasis. In the interest of applying the least possible astigmatic treatment in a specific situation where the refractive cylinder and the corneal astigmatism are quite disparate, the clinician might choose an emphasis where the TIA is at its least possible magnitude (shortest length), leaving the astigmatic situation largely unchanged.

Other tips of this type are included in my rules of thumb. I hope you find that, when it comes to applying the Alpins Method in clinical situations, less is sometimes more than enough, and can result in great satisfaction for both patient and physician.

REFERENCES

1. Alpins N. Astigmatism analysis by the Alpins method. *J Cataract Refract Surg.* 2001;27(1):31-49.
2. Alpins N, Stamatelatos G. Customized photoastigmatic refractive keratectomy using combined topographic and refractive data for myopia and astigmatism in eyes with forme fruste and mild keratoconus. *J Cataract Refract Surg.* 2007;33(4):591-602.
3. Alpins NA. New method of targeting vectors to treat astigmatism. *J Cataract Refract Surg.* 1997;23(1):65-75.
4. Alpins NA, Stamatelatos G. Combined wavefront and topography approach to refractive surgery treatments. In: Wang M, ed. *Corneal Topography in the Wavefront Era: A Guide for Clinical Application.* Thorofare, NJ: SLACK Incorporated; 2006:139-143.
5. Alpins NA. Wavefront technology: a new advance that fails to answer old questions on corneal vs. refractive astigmatism correction. *J Refract Surg.* 2002;18(6):737-739.
6. Walsh MJ. Is the future of refractive surgery based on corneal topography or wavefront? Ocular Surgery News Web site. http://www.healio.com/ophthalmology/refractive-surgery/news/print/ocular-surgery-news/%7Bdf8c4698-b178-47f7-83cb-b3c890916b7f%7D/is-the-future-of-refractive-surgery-based-on-corneal-topography-or-wavefront. Published August 1, 2000. Accessed August 9, 2014.

7. Alpins N, Stamatelatos G. Clinical outcomes of laser in situ keratomileusis using combined topography and refractive wavefront treatments for myopic astigmatism. *J Cataract Refract Surg.* 2008;34(8):1250-1259.

8. Alpins NA, Schmid L. Combining vector planning with wavefront analysis to optimize laser in-situ keratomileusis outcomes. In: Krueger RR, Applegate RA, MacRae SM, eds. *Wavefront Customized Visual Correction: The Quest for Super Vision II.* Thorofare, NJ: SLACK Incorporated; 2004:317-328.

9. Kugler L, Cohen I, Haddad W, Wang MX. Efficacy of laser in situ keratomileusis in correcting anterior and non-anterior corneal astigmatism: comparative study. *J Cataract Refract Surg.* 2010;36(10):1745-1752.

10. Qian YS, Huang J, Liu R, et al. Influence of internal optical astigmatism on the correction of myopic astigmatism by LASIK. *J Refract Surg.* 2011;27(12):863-868.

11. Lackner B, Schmidinger G, Pieh S, Funovics MA, Skorpik C. Repeatability and reproducibility of central corneal thickness measurement with Pentacam, Orbscan, and ultrasound. *Optom Vis Sci.* 2005;82(10):892-899.

12. Wang L, Mahmoud AM, Anderson BL, Koch DD, Roberts CJ. Total corneal power estimation: ray tracing method versus gaussian optics formula. *Invest Ophthalmol Vis Sci.* 2011;52(3):1716-22.

13. Yaylali V, Kaufman SC, Thompson HW. Corneal thickness measurements with the Orbscan Topography System and ultrasonic pachymetry. *J Cataract Refract Surg.* 1997;23(9):1345-1350.

14. Alpins N, Ong JK, Stamatelatos G. New method of quantifying corneal topographic astigmatism that corresponds with manifest refractive cylinder. *J Cataract Refract Surg.* 2012;38(11):1978-1988.

15. Alpins NA, Ong JKY, Stamatelatos G. Corneal topographic astigmatism (CorT) to quantify total corneal astigmatism. *J Refract Surg.* 2015;31(3):182-186.

16. Koch DD, Ali SF, Weikert MP, Shirayama M, Jenkins R, Wang L. Contribution of posterior corneal astigmatism to total corneal astigmatism. *J Cataract Refract Surg.* 2012;38(12):2080-2087.

17. Koch DD, Jenkins RB, Weikert MP, Yeu E, Wang L. Correcting astigmatism with toric intraocular lenses: effect of posterior corneal astigmatism. *J Cataract Refract Surg.* 2013;39(12):1803-1809.

18. Alpins N. Combining wavefront and topography data [letter]. *J Cataract Refract Surg.* 2005;31(4):646-647.

19. Alpins NA. A new method of analyzing vectors for changes in astigmatism. *J Cataract Refract Surg.* 1993;19(4):524-533.

20. Alpins N, Stamatelatos G. *Asymmetrical surgical treatment using vector planning.* In: Wang M, ed. Thorofare, NJ: SLACK Incorporated; 2008:263-268.

21. Alpins NA. Vector analysis of astigmatism changes by flattening, steepening, and torque. *J Cataract Refract Surg.* 1997;23(10):1503-1514.

22. Alpins NA. Treatment of irregular astigmatism. *J Cataract Refract Surg.* 1998;24(5):634-646.

23. Alpins NA. Corneal versus refractive astigmatism: integrated analysis. *Ocular Surgery News.* June 15, 1999:44.

24. Alpins NA. Flattening, steepening, and torque are crucial points in astigmatism surgery. *Ocular Surgery News.* June 1, 1999:19.

25. Alpins NA. Vector analysis of astigmatism correction: the Alpins method. *Ocular Surgery News.* May 15, 1999:14.

26. Alpins NA. The treatment of irregular astigmatism. *Ocular Surgery News.* July 1, 1999:6.

27. Alpins NA. Topographic disparity: a useful new measure of irregular astigmatism. *Ocular Surgery News.* July 15, 1999:8.

28. Alpins NA. The treatment of irregular astigmatism. *Ocular Surgery News.* July 1, 1999:6.

29. Alpins NA, Goggin M. Practical astigmatism analysis for refractive outcomes in cataract and refractive surgery. *Surv Ophthalmol.* 2004;49(1):109-122.

30. Darwin C. *The Origin of Species.* London, England: John Murray; 1859.

31. Stear J. The incomprehensible creationist: the Darwin "eye" quote revisited.. No Answers in Genesis! Web site. http://www.noanswersingenesis.org.au/darwin_eye_quote_revisited.htm. Updated 16 May 2005. Accessed November 5, 2015.

32. National Portrait Gallery Web site. http://www.npg.org.uk/collections/search/use-this-image.php?mkey=mw01728. Accessed June 15, 2017.

33. Evolution of the eye. Wikipedia Web site. https://en.wikipedia.org/wiki/Evolution_of_the_eye. Accessed November 5, 2015.

34. Lamb TD. Evolution of the eye [subscription or payment required]. Scientific American Web site. http://www.scientificamerican.com/article/evolution-of-the-eye. Accessed November 5, 2015.

35. Nilsson DE, Pelger S. A pessimistic estimate of the time required for an eye to evolve. *Proc Biol Sci.* 1994;256(1345):53-58.

36. Alpins NA, Terry CM. Astigmatism: LASIK, LASEK, and PRK. In: Roy FH, Arzabe CW, eds. *Master Techniques in Cataract and Refractive Surgery.* Thorofare, NJ: SLACK Incorporated; 2004:151-160.

37. Boyle EL. Experts differ on corneal astigmatism correction in cataract surgery. Eyeworld. Feburary, 2013.

38. Baldwin WR, Mills D. A longitudinal study of corneal astigmatism and total astigmatism. *Am J Optom Physiol Opt.* 1981;58(3):206-211.

Chapter 15

Not Everyone Has Regular Astigmatism
The Hemidivisional Solution

A Quick Review of Previous Lessons

The cornerstone of the Alpins Method involves a separate and independent evaluation of the subjective experience of vision (refraction) and the objective measurement of corneal shape (topography, tomography, keratometry, etc). This is the founding principle—and, originally, a philosophical stumbling block—from which all other elements of the Alpins Method were derived.

We know that astigmatism distorts vision (Figure 15-1). We also know that astigmatism relates both to eye-brain perception and the culminating pattern of light from its path through the anterior cornea through all physiologic elements of the eye back to the retina. Yet refractive procedures such as laser in situ keratomileusis (LASIK) are restricted to the anterior cornea.

Previous chapters have taught us a number of lessons:

- Simply sculpting a refractive correction onto the anterior surface of the cornea does not appear to be an optimal approach, in some cases leading to greater postoperative corneal astigmatism and lower-than-expected visual acuity[1-4] (Chapter 3).
- Ocular residual astigmatism (ORA) represents the absolute lower limit of astigmatism possible to attain in any given eye, even if the procedure is done perfectly[1,5,6] (Chapter 9).
- Use of corneal topographic astigmatism (CorT)[7] anterior (a measure of corneal topographic astigmatism) and CorT total[8] (a measure of CorT also employing posterior corneal astigmatism) provides a more accurate assessment of manifest refractive cylinder than other methods—for example, keratometry, simulated keratometry (SimK), corneal wavefront, and paraxial curvature matching (Chapter 12).
- The Vector Planning approach optimizes both corneal and refractive astigmatism[9-11] (Chapter 13).

Alpins N. *Practical Astigmatism:*
Planning and Analysis (pp 123-126).
© 2018 SLACK Incorporated.

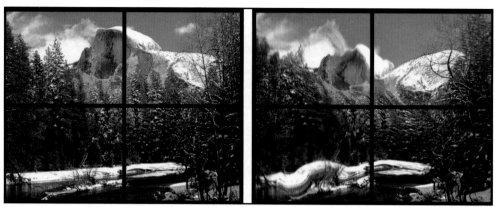

Figure 15-1. A patient with no astigmatism can appreciate an undistorted view (left), while someone with astigmatism may see a distorted image (right).

We also know that many patients have corneal maps that look something like that shown in Figure 15-2—patients with irregular astigmatism.

Irregular astigmatism exists when the two steepest astigmatism meridians of opposite hemidivisions are (1) other than 180° apart (nonorthogonal); (2) the magnitude of astigmatism differs between hemidivisions (asymmetric); or (3) both conditions exist (nonorthogonal asymmetric).[12]

We have discussed in previous chapters the idea of providing optimal treatment separately to the corneal hemidivisions. At this writing, no lasers are available that can accomplish this. Still, we have described a method to treat irregular astigmatism; the approach incorporates vector calculation to arrive at an "average" treatment based on the disparate measurements of the two hemidivisions.[12]

THE CORNEAL SPLIT

The calculation of CorT is included in the iASSORT (Alpins Statistical System for Ophthalmic Refractive surgery Techniques) software and is programmed into leading corneal topography and tomography devices. The Alpins Method at this point has been developed to consider the two hemidivisions of a cornea with irregular astigmatism. The program automatically divides the eye into two hemidivisions based on the nature of the irregular astigmatism in a specific patient.

It is important to understand that the use of hemidivisions is arbitrary—that one could divide (and base calculations on) quadrants of the cornea, or even splitting the cornea into 360 separate 1° "omnidivisions." The latter undoubtedly exceeds any current exigency, but remains a tantalizing future option.

Also, the corneal "split" between hemidivisions does not have to lie on the horizontal 0°-to-180° axis, as implied by the juxtaposition of a polar diagram on a corneal map, such as shown in Figure 15-2. In fact, for the purpose of calculating a CorT anterior and CorT total for each hemidivision, the cornea can be divided in half at any axis. The iASSORT

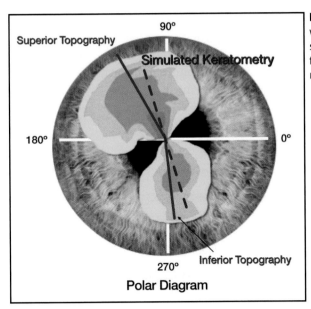

Figure 15-2. A corneal map of a patient with irregular astigmatism demonstrates the familiar skewed bowtie configuration, which is both nonorthogonal and asymmetric.

program selects this split based on the flat meridian of the CorT anterior or CorT total (if available). And this is the "hemidivisional solution."

For the calculation of CorT anterior and CorT total, all visible Placido rings are used. Prior to CorT, we chose the 5-mm ring, as the 7-mm ring is sometimes obscured by the eyelid and the 3-mm ring does not contain enough data. In either event, the program selects the dividing meridian between hemidivisions and assigns one half as "superior" and the other as "inferior"; again, this dividing meridian can be on any axis. (Programming included in corneal topographers currently does not make a distinction between hemidivisions in calculating CorT; this is only possible using the iASSORT software).

We choose the average of the flat meridia when we use CorT; thus, the flattening treatment is done on the steep meridian 90° away. The CorT anterior is actually the vectorial sum of the CorTsup (superior) and the CorTinf (inferior) and the CorT total is the vectorial sum of the CorTsup total and the CorTinf total.

A CORNEAL TOPOGRAPHIC ASTIGMATISM FOR ALL CORNEAS

As discussed in Chapter 12, CorT (anterior and total) provides a consistent measure of corneal astigmatism whether regular or irregular. A separate CorT calculation is made for each hemidivision, which generates a magnitude value and a meridian value for each half of the cornea. When these calculations are added vectorially, the result is a CorT for the entire cornea. When these values are subtracted vectorially, the surgeon can determine the dioptric difference of one half of the cornea from the other half, called topographic disparity (TD).[7,12] TD, which is related to ORA, is further described in Chapter 16. A TD > 1 D is considered significant, and incorporating the Vector Planning approach in the treatment paradigm becomes essential to minimize the corneal astigmatism remaining postoperatively.

All this evokes some fascinating treatment possibilities, which are further discussed in Chapter 17: the "regularization" of irregular astigmatism, using the "optimal" treatment I have described, and the use of hemidivisional laser treatments that promise better visual acuity with no change in spectacle refraction. Future refinements in technology will make this analytic methodology invaluable. Stay tuned!

REFERENCES

1. Alpins NA. New method of targeting vectors to treat astigmatism. *J Cataract Refract Surg.* 1997;23(1):65-75.

2. Qian YS, Huang J, Liu R, et al. Influence of internal optical astigmatism on the correction of myopic astigmatism by LASIK. *J Refract Surg.* 2011;27(12):863-868.

3. Kugler L, Cohen I, Haddad W, Wang MX. Efficacy of laser in situ keratomileusis in correcting anterior and non-anterior corneal astigmatism: comparative study. *J Cataract Refract Surg.* 2010;36(10):1745-1752.

4. Frings A, Katz T, Steinberg J, Druchkiv V, Richard G, Linke SJ. Ocular residual astigmatism: effects of demographic and ocular parameters in myopic laser in situ keratomileusis. *J Cataract Refract Surg.* 2014;40(2):232-238.

5. Alpins NA. A new method of analyzing vectors for changes in astigmatism. *J Cataract Refract Surg.* 1993;19(4):524-533.

6. Alpins N. Astigmatism analysis by the Alpins method. *J Cataract Refract Surg.* 2001;27(1):31-49.

7. Alpins N, Ong JK, Stamatelatos G. New method of quantifying corneal topographic astigmatism that corresponds with manifest refractive cylinder. *J Cataract Refract Surg.* 2012;38(11):1978-1988.

8. Alpins NA, Ong JKY, Stamatelatos G. Corneal topographic astigmatism (CorT) to quantify total corneal astigmatism. *J Refract Surg.* 2015;31(3):182-186.

9. Alpins N. Combining wavefront and topography data [letter]. *J Cataract Refract Surg.* 2005;31(4):646-647.

10. Alpins N, Stamatelatos G. Customized photoastigmatic refractive keratectomy using combined topographic and refractive data for myopia and astigmatism in eyes with forme fruste and mild keratoconus. *J Cataract Refract Surg.* 2007;33(4):591-602.

11. Alpins N, Stamatelatos G. Clinical outcomes of laser in situ keratomileusis using combined topography and refractive wavefront treatments for myopic astigmatism. *J Cataract Refract Surg.* 2008;34(8):1250-1259.

12. Alpins NA. Treatment of irregular astigmatism. *J Cataract Refract Surg.* 1998;24(5):634-646.

Chapter 16

Topographic Disparity
Quantifying Corneal Irregularity

A NATURAL EXTENSION OF THE ALPINS METHOD

The Alpins Method has become standard in reporting clinical studies that include astigmatism outcomes in refractive surgery.[1-5] In the years following my initial description of the Alpins Method,[6] a number of refinements and nuanced applications naturally occurred to me—for example, ocular residual astigmatism (ORA) and the nonzero target[7-9] (Chapters 9 and 5, respectively); flattening, steepening, and torque[10,11] (Chapter 8); managing "refractive surprises" after toric intraocular lens implantation[12,13] (Chapters 10 and 11); the concepts of corneal topographic astigmatism (CorT)[14] and CorT total,[15] (Chapter 12); and the Vector Planning approach in patients having astigmatism. Use of the Alpins Method and the Vector Planning approach for patients with irregular astigmatism (Chapter 15) was a natural extension.

A key calculation in evaluating irregular astigmatism is the topographic disparity (TD). Although lasers are not yet available that can separately and systematically treat the two hemidivisions of a cornea with irregular astigmatism, understanding TD has immediate clinical importance, and undoubtedly will figure into future treatment options. Chapter 17 describes a number of potential future treatment approaches in patients with irregular astigmatism.

A CALCULATION USING THE iASSORT PROGRAM

TD is calculated with the iASSORT (Alpins Statistical System for Ophthalmic Refractive surgery Techniques) program using corneal measurements that can be generated by many currently available topography/tomography devices. It is important that the practitioner uses the same approach preoperatively as postoperatively; for example, the use of preoperative CorT should be compared against postoperative CorT, maintaining an apples-to-apples assessment of the patient over time.

As described in Chapters 12 and 15, the programming in iASSORT automatically selects the flat meridian of the CorT to divide the cornea and calculate the TD between

Alpins N. *Practical Astigmatism:*
Planning and Analysis (pp 127-131).
© 2018 SLACK Incorporated.

Figure 16-1. TD is calculated using a 720° double-angle vector diagram (right). Conversion to a polar diagram can then be shown superimposed over the eye (left). The length of the TD line quantifies the amount of irregularity. Certain orientations of the TD in the polar diagram may be clinically beneficial, but more study of this is needed.

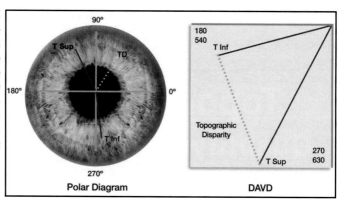

the resulting hemidivisions. For the calculation of CorT anterior and CorT total, all visible rings are used in each hemidivision. Prior to our use of CorT, we chose the 5-mm ring, as the 7-mm ring is sometimes obscured by the eyelid. The program selects the dividing meridian between hemidivisions and assigns one half as "superior" and the other as "inferior" depending on the divider's position. A separate CorT calculation is made for each hemidivision, which generates a magnitude value and a meridian value for each half of the cornea. When these calculations are added vectorially, the result is a CorT for the entire cornea (CorT anterior or CorT total depending on what data are available from the topographic device). When these values are subtracted vectorially, the surgeon can determine the dioptric difference as well as the meridional difference of one half of the cornea from the other half—the TD.[14,16]

THE ROAD TO PERFECTION

The TD in a patient with irregular astigmatism is a necessary measure for "perfect" treatment—that is, "reduction and regularization"—as described in Chapter 17. Although current laser technology does not offer systematic, discrete hemidivisional treatment in a cornea with irregular astigmatism, TD as an analytic tool provides much insight. TD allows us to quantify irregularity and its axis,[16-18] and is related to a number of variables found in irregular corneas.[13,19]

The TD is calculated as the dioptric distance between the displays of superior and inferior topographic dioptric steep meridian values on a 720° double-angle vector diagram (DAVD). The TD quantifies both the nonorthogonal and asymmetrical component of corneal irregularity as a single dioptric magnitude value with an axis. Furthermore, the TD is a standardized parameter of corneal irregularity across most topography/tomography devices, so that the TD from one device can be compared with the TD from another. Figure 16-1 shows the DAVD together with a polar diagram; the polar diagram superimposed over the cornea provides a clinical idea of the magnitude and orientation of the irregularity in this sample patient.

How prevalent is a "significant" level of TD? In a group of 100 consecutive patients with virgin corneas, we found a mean TD of 1.10 D ± 0.08 D (range 0.04 to 4.70 D), and a TD > 1.00 D in 43 patients[16] (Figure 16-2). Thus, TD is a factor that should be considered in almost half of your refractive surgery patients.

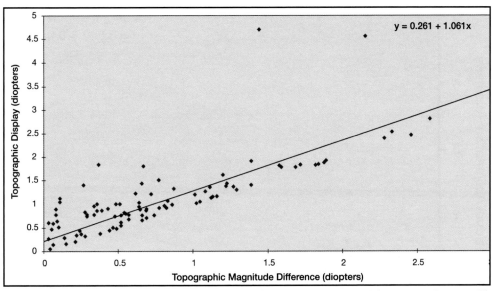

Figure 16-2. In a group of 100 consecutive patients, the mean TD was 1.10 D (range 0.04 D to 4.70 D). TD exceeded 1.00 D in 43 eyes.[16] (Reprinted from *Journal of Cataract & Refractive Surgery*, 24/5, Alpins NA, Treatment of irregular astigmatism, 13, Copyright 1998, with permission from Elsevier.)

We also showed a statistically significant relationship between TD and 15:

- The difference between superior and inferior topographic magnitude values
- The angle of the topographic nonorthogonal astigmatism—that is, the angle subtended between the upper (superior) and lower (inferior) meridians of astigmatism
- The meridian of simulated keratometry (SimK)

There also is a direct proportional relationship between increasing ORA and TD; that is, the greater the TD, the greater the ORA (Figure 16-3).[16] This was encountered in a study we performed on patients with forme fruste and mild keratoconus[7] where a higher-than-average ORA (1.34 D) was found due to a higher amount of keratoconus-related corneal irregularity as calculated using the TD (2.32 D).

As with all treatments described in this book, when treating irregular corneas, it is important to consider the topography values in the treatment plan, as treatment based solely on the manifest refraction or the wavefront aberrometry second-order cylinder can leave the cornea with excess avoidable astigmatism.

THE ALPINS METHOD IN MANAGING PATIENT EXPECTATIONS

In recent years, the importance of the Alpins Method in studying and reporting the results of refractive surgery has become apparent.[1-5] Researchers finally have a useful, comprehensive, common language in their approach to astigmatism. This higher level of care also applies to the many patients with irregular astigmatism, whose potential treatment approaches are described in Chapter 17.

Currently, the increased understanding afforded by the Alpins Method has an impact mainly on the management of patient expectations. If the TD is more than

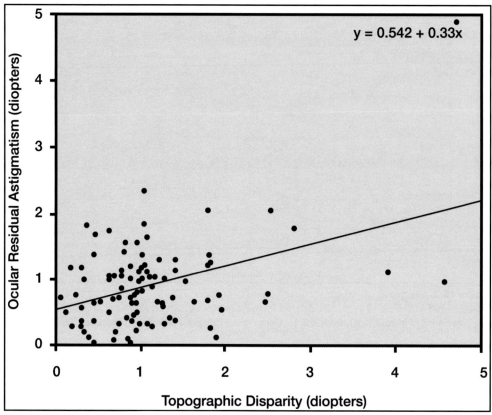

Figure 16-3. Ocular residual astigmatism magnitude vs topographic disparity magnitude in 100 consecutive patients ($P < .0001$).[16] A direct relationship between the two measures is evident. (Reprinted from *Journal of Cataract & Refractive Surgery*, 24/5, Alpins NA, Treatment of irregular astigmatism, 13, Copyright 1998, with permission from Elsevier.)

1.00 D, then it is advisable to calculate the ORA, as the ORA in most cases will also be high. Therefore, It is critically important that the treatment paradigm include both corneal and refractive measures of astigmatism. In this way, patients with high TD and/or high ORA can be advised that they likely will remain with some astigmatism after laser vision correction. These patients can also be told that the Vector Planning approach, using both corneal and refractive values, will maximally reduce the amount of total astigmatism postoperatively.

TD may also be used as an early detector of keratoconus due to the asymmetry between the superior and inferior cornea in these patients.[7,20] Furthermore, a reduction in best corrected vision may indicate a high TD, which should be calculated as confirmation. Studies are required to understand if there is any significance in the orientation of the TD and whether some orientations are more favorable than others to visual outcomes of surgery.

REFERENCES

1. Author Information Pack. American Academy of Ophthalmology Web site. https://www.elsevier.com/wps/find/journaldescription.cws_home/620418?generatepdf=true. Accessed January 19, 2016.

2. Information for Authors. American Society of Cataract and Refractive Surgery Web site. http://www.jcrsjournal.org/content/authorinfo#info. Accessed September 1, 2016.

3. Reinstein DZ, Archer TJ, Randleman JB. JRS standard for reporting astigmatism outcomes of refractive surgery [editorial]. *J Refract Surg*. 2014;30(10):654-659.

4. Reinstein DZ, Randleman JB, Archer TJ, et al. JRS standard for reporting outcomes of intraocular lens based refractive surgery. *J Refract Surg*. 2017;33(4):218-222.

5. Reinstein DZ, Archer TJ, Srinivasan S, Mamalis N, Kohnen T, Dupps Jr WJ, Randleman JB. Standard for reporting refractive outcomes of intraocular lens-based refractive surgery. *Journal Cataract Refract Surg*. 2017;43(4):435-439.

6. Alpins NA. A new method of analyzing vectors for changes in astigmatism. *J Cataract Refract Surg*. 1993;19(4):524-533.

7. Alpins N, Stamatelatos G. Customized photoastigmatic refractive keratectomy using combined topographic and refractive data for myopia and astigmatism in eyes with forme fruste and mild keratoconus. *J Cataract Refract Surg*. 2007;33(4):591-602.

8. Alpins N, Stamatelatos G. Clinical outcomes of laser in situ keratomileusis using combined topography and refractive wavefront treatments for myopic astigmatism. *J Cataract Refract Surg*. 2008;34(8):1250-1259.

9. Alpins NA, Tabin GC, Adams LM, Aldred GF, Kent DG, Taylor HR. Refractive versus corneal changes after photorefractive keratectomy for astigmatism. *J Refract Surg*. 1998;14(4):386-396.

10. Alpins NA. Vector analysis of astigmatism changes by flattening, steepening, and torque. *J Cataract Refract Surg*. 1997;23(10):1503-1514.

11. Alpins NA. Flattening, steepening, and torque are crucial points in astigmatism surgery. *Ocular Surgery News*. June 1, 1999:19.

12. Alpins N, Ong JK, Stamatelatos G. Refractive surprise after toric intraocular lens implantation: graph analysis. *J Cataract Refract Surg*. 2014;40(2):283-294.

13. Alpins N, Stamatelatos G. Correcting refractive surprises after toric IOL implantation. *Cataract & Refractive Surgery Today Europe*. 2014;20-22.

14. Alpins N, Ong JK, Stamatelatos G. New method of quantifying corneal topographic astigmatism that corresponds with manifest refractive cylinder. *J Cataract Refract Surg*. 2012;38(11):1978-1988.

15. Alpins NA, Ong JKY, Stamatelatos G. Corneal topographic astigmatism (CorT) to quantify total corneal astigmatism. *J Refract Surg*. 2015;31(3):182-186.

16. Alpins NA. Treatment of irregular astigmatism. *J Cataract Refract Surg*. 1998;24(5):634-646.

17. Alpins N, Stamatelatos G. *Asymmetrical surgical treatment using vector planning*. In: Wang M, ed. Thorofare, NJ: SLACK Incorporated; 2008:263-268.

18. Goggin M, Alpins N, Schmid LM. Management of irregular astigmatism. *Curr Opin Ophthalmol*. 2000;11(4):260-266.

19. Alpins N, Ong JKY, Stamatelatos G. Corneal coupling of astigmatism applied to incisional and ablative surgery. *J Cataract Refract Surg*. 2014;40:1813-1827.

20. Martinez-Abad A, Pinero DP, Ruiz-Fortes P, Artola A. Evaluation of the diagnostic ability of vector parameters characterizing the corneal astigmatism and regularity in clinical and subclinical keratoconus. *Cont Lens Anterior Eye*. 2017;40(2):88-96.

Chapter 17

The Perfect Treatment
Reduction and Regularization

THE ALPINS METHOD × 2

In previous chapters I described how the essence of the Alpins Method is captured by a golf putt (Figure 17-1). The intended effect of the astigmatism surgery (the path from the ball to the cup) is the target induced astigmatism vector (TIA).[1,2] The actual putt (the path the ball takes when hit) corresponds to the surgically induced astigmatism vector (SIA).[3] The second putt needed to hit the cup corresponds to the difference vector (DV), or the amount and orientation of the astigmatism treatment required to achieve the original target. A double-angle vector diagram (DAVD) of these three fundamental vectors is shown in Figure 17-2; these vectors and their relationships comprise the essence of the Alpins Method.

Chapters 15 and 16 describe the use of the Alpins Method in patients with irregular astigmatism. In essence, the patient with irregular astigmatism is assessed in the same way as a patient with regular astigmatism; however, the division of the cornea into 2 hemidivisions comprising the irregularity requires that our figurative golfer confront 2 separate situations—that is, astigmatism on separate axes (nonorthogonal) and/or of differing magnitudes (asymmetric). In the case of a patient with irregular astigmatism, each hemidivision also has a separate TIA, connoting treatment beyond the scope of current laser technology for a single pass.

However, such will not always be the case; lasers will one day be available to routinely treat in the one process the separate hemidivisions of the irregular cornea. This chapter discusses the controlled manipulation of corneal shape by asymmetrical surgical treatment of the differing nonorthogonal and/or asymmetrical hemidivisions of the cornea, allowing for the achievement of any desired corneal shape[4,5] (Figure 17-3).

Alpins N. *Practical Astigmatism:
Planning and Analysis* (pp 133-140).
© 2018 SLACK Incorporated.

Figure 17-1. The basics of the Alpins Method are neatly conveyed by a golf putt. The intended effect of the astigmatism surgery (the path from the ball to the cup) is the TIA.[1,2] The actual putt (the path the ball takes when hit) corresponds to the SIA.[3] The second putt needed to hit the cup corresponds to the DV, or the amount and orientation of the astigmatism treatment required to achieve the original target. The relationships that exist among these three fundamental vectors (TIA, SIA, and DV) provide helpful indices that form the foundation of the Alpins Method.

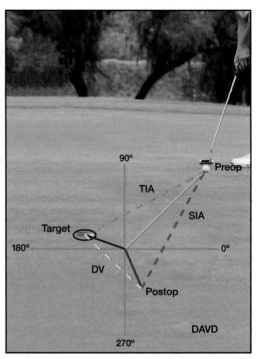

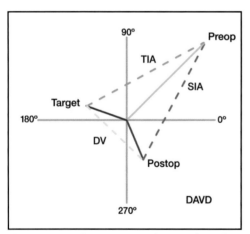

Figure 17-2. The TIA, SIA, and DV are based on the golf putt shown in Figure 17-1. The TIA, SIA, and DV are calculated from (1) the patient's preoperative astigmatism; (2) the targeted astigmatism the surgeon plans to achieve; and (3) the actual achieved effect of the surgery. In patients with irregular astigmatism, similar analyses are conducted separately for each hemidivision of the cornea.

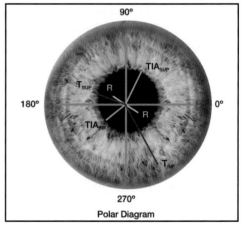

Figure 17-3. A polar diagram is superimposed over the eye, showing the optimal asymmetric treatment (surgical vector parameters) calculated for each hemidivision in an eye with irregular astigmatism. Abbreviations: INF, inferior; R, refractive astigmatism; SUP, superior; T, topographic astigmatism; TIA, targeted induced astigmatism vector.

THREE BASIC APPROACHES TO TREATING IRREGULAR ASTIGMATISM

This chapter deals with 3 basic approaches to irregular astigmatism:

1. *Optimal treatment of the hemidivisions*—As with the "optimal approach" described in Chapter 6, the closer the target corneal astigmatism is to an against-the-rule (ATR) orientation, the more emphasis is placed on correcting the corneal astigmatism. This approach favors a postoperative with-the-rule (WTR) astigmatism, and is based on what appears to be a greater neurophysiologic tolerance of or preference for WTR astigmatism. Optimal treatment of each hemidivision means that the superior hemidivision can have, for example, a 40% emphasis on topography and a 60% emphasis on refraction, while the inferior hemidivision can have a 30% emphasis on topography and 70% emphasis on refraction. The closer the resulting corneal astigmatism is to being WTR, the more it can be left on the cornea.

2. *Regularization of the cornea*—This treatment attempts to produce symmetrical orthogonal topography with no change in refractive astigmatism. Patients could then be expected to have a better quality of vision without having to change their current spectacles if that is their preference. This approach would allow the creation of "see-better" clinics, which have been discussed by many investigators for many years. For this type of refractive surgery, laser astigmatic treatments (that is, the TIA) are identical but opposite; that is, laser treatments are at right angles to each other on a polar display or 180° away on a DAVD. The skewed "bowtie" as seen on a corneal map would be straightened and symmetrical.

3. *Regularization and reduction by changing topography of one or both hemimeridians*—What might be called "the perfect treatment," regularization and reduction refers to treatment that aligns irregular astigmatism, converting a nonorthogonal to an orthogonal orientation, and simultaneously reducing the magnitude of astigmatism, seeking a spherical equivalent of zero. This approach can involve an astigmatic change to only one hemidivision of the cornea with no change in the other topographic hemimeridian is targeted. Another intuitive method to achieve an orthogonal and symmetrical cornea is to topographically target the refractive astigmatism magnitude and axis in both hemidivisions of the cornea. This will result in a net reduction in the ocular residual astigmatism (ORA) and minimize the corneal astigmatism due to the decrease in the difference between topography and refraction in each hemidivision.

The ASSORT (Alpins Statistical System for Ophthalmic Refractive surgery Techniques) program readily calculates these treatments based on refractive values and corneal astigmatism as measured by all available technologies. The practitioner should simply remember to use the same technology in following any individual patient to avoid instrument-specific or technique-specific measurement differences. It is also important to recall that all of these calculated treatment approaches have a TIA that extends to the vector of ORA on a DAVD when treating optimally. This means that, no matter which emphasis is chosen—100% topography, 100% refraction, or any combination of the 2 equaling 100%—the minimum amount of astigmatism (the ORA) remains on both hemidivisions. Remember, the maximum correction of astigmatism is achieved when the remaining astigmatism is at its minimum and is equal to the ORA.[6,7] The concurrent regularization of the minimal corneal astigmatism remaining makes it the perfect treatment.

WITH-THE-RULE VERSUS AGAINST-THE-RULE ASTIGMATISM

As discussed in Chapter 9, ORA exists in any eye in which refractive and corneal astigmatism are of unequal magnitude and/or axis. In a study of 100 consecutive eyes,[6] I found that the magnitude of topographic astigmatism exceeded refractive astigmatism in 59 patients; refractive astigmatism was greater in the remaining 41. A minority of patients had < 10° of angular separation between topographic and refractive measurements; many had 10° or greater separation (up to almost 80°). Interestingly, for patients with topographical meridia closer to 90°, the magnitude of topographical astigmatism exceeded that of refractive astigmatism; and for those with topographical meridia closer to 180°, refractive astigmatism had the greater magnitude value. This finding supports the widely-held idea that people have a greater optical tolerance for WTR astigmatism.

WTR astigmatism tends to change to ATR astigmatism with increasing age; that is, younger patients tend towards WTR astigmatism and older patients to ATR astigmatism.[8] WTR astigmatism is more common than ATR astigmatism.[9] In general, WTR astigmatism is visually more favorable than ATR astigmatism, and oblique astigmatism is the least favorable.[5] The preference for WTR astigmatism in distance vision dates back to Javal's rule, published in 1890.[10]

RECONCILING MEASURES OF CORNEAL AND REFRACTIVE IRREGULARITY

We have discussed in previous chapters the idea of providing optimal treatment separately to the corneal hemidivisions. At this writing, no lasers exist that can accomplish this with one treatment session. Still, we have described a method using existing laser technology to treat irregular astigmatism; this approach incorporates vector calculation to arrive at an "average" treatment that incorporates the disparate measurements of the 2 hemidivisions.[4]

Any method either to "minimize" or "regularize" a cornea with irregular astigmatism faces substantial complexities. To correct such astigmatism, it is not enough to suggest that a methodical refraction can resolve the differences. The refractive cylinder measures, not only the corneal astigmatism, but all the optical interfaces of the eye and the interpretation of the image by the cerebral cortex. Also, there is no mechanism to reconcile which of the 2 hemimeridians—either in regular or irregular astigmatism—may have been resolved with the manifest refractive astigmatism.

When the TIA between the 2 hemidivisions of an eye with irregular astigmatism differs, a summation of the TIAs (TIA_{NET}) or vectorial average needs to be calculated to determine the combined effect on refractive astigmatism. This TIA_{NET} is then applied to the common refractive astigmatism value of the 2 hemidivisions to determine the expected average refractive astigmatism value for the whole eye.

Looking at the astigmatic treatments applied to the refraction for the options described previously:
- *Reduction of corneal astigmatism by optimal treatment of each hemidivision—* When the astigmatic treatment between the 2 hemidivisions differs, the change in the refractive astigmatism is the vectorial average of the 2 hemidivisions (Figure 17-4).

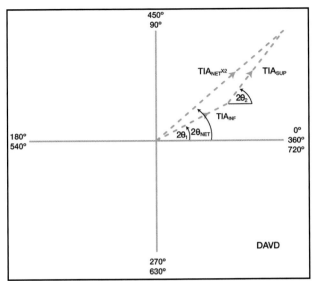

Figure 17-4. The 2 treatment vectors (TIA$_{SUP}$ and TIA$_{INF}$) are averaged by adding 1 to the other, resulting in a TIA$_{NETx2}$. This TIA$_{NETx2}$ must now be divided by 2 and the orientation of it halved when converted to a polar diagram.

- *Regularization of the cornea*—The topographical astigmatism of the 2 hemi-meridians can be targeted to coincide in both magnitude and meridian so that the average treatment has no net effect on the refractive astigmatism (Figure 17-5).

- *Shifting one topography hemimeridian to achieve an orthogonal, symmetrical cornea*—The total astigmatism treatment here (TIA$_{NET}$) that is applied to the refractive astigmatism is half that of the single treatment, regardless of which hemimeridian was moved. The minimum treatment to regularize the cornea is equal to the topographic disparity (TD) (Figure 17-6).

- *Shifting both topography hemimeridians to target the refractive astigmatism magnitude and axis*—The refractive astigmatism induced by the net TIA change will shift (Figure 17-7). The resultant ORA of both hemidivisions will be reduced and equal.

- *Reduction and regularization treating both corneal hemimeridians*—There are 2 options here: (1) to reduce the corneal astigmatism and then regularize it; or (2) to regularize the corneal astigmatism and then reduce it.

Future technology may enable measurement of separate refractive errors for each hemidivision of the cornea by devices such as aberrometers. This would potentially improve visual outcomes further by an accurate measurement of second-order pre- and postoperative readings. Additionally, regularization of the topographic targets can be achieved after this maximum reduction of the astigmatism by targeting the common refraction, and hence, reducing the prevailing ORA. Multiple variations to this maximum reduction and regularization of astigmatism are possible, giving the surgeon the means to change the corneal shape to that desired. These include achieving orthogonal symmetrical astigmatism without changing the refractive astigmatism as described above, hence, achieving a summated TIA$_{NET}$ of 0.00 D.

As many as 40% of "normal" corneas with an astigmatic refractive error can be said to have primary irregular astigmatism.[11] Irregularity may exist across the corneal hemidivision as a difference in dioptric magnitude (asymmetry) or orientation (nonor-

Figure 17-5. The 2 astigmatic treatment vectors for each half of the cornea are equal in magnitude but opposite in direction on a DAVD. The resultant treatment TIA$_{NETx2}$ is now zero and the refractive astigmatism will remain unaltered while regularizing the irregularity.

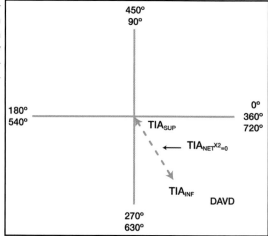

Figure 17-6. There is only one astigmatic treatment in this option to treat irregular astigmatism, as only one of the topographic hemimeridians is changed. This single TIA is still divided by 2 to obtain the net effective treatment that will be applied to the refractive astigmatism.

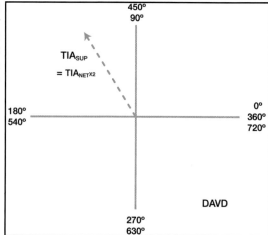

Figure 17-7. Summation of superior and inferior treatment vectors determine the net TIA, which is then halved in magnitude and axis on a polar diagram.

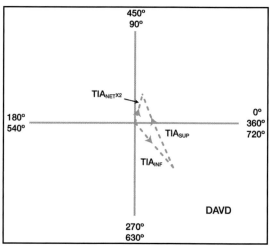

thogonal) or both. I have described TD as a tool for quantifying corneal irregularity.[4] TD is the dioptric separation between the 2 corneal hemidivisions as shown on a 720° DAVD, described in Chapter 16. TD > 1.00 D is found in 44% of eyes with treatable astigmatism.[4,11]

There is a direct proportional relationship between increasing ORA and TD; the greater the TD, the greater the ORA.[4] It is therefore of utmost importance when treating irregular corneas, that the topography values for astigmatism be incorporated into the treatment plan using the Vector Planning approach, as treatment based on the manifest refraction or the wavefront aberrometry cylinder alone can leave the cornea with excess avoidable astigmatism.

PLAN THE WORK AND WORK THE PLAN

As described, the Vector Planning approach can be applied to formulate separate surgical plans and unique TIA values for each hemidivision. Inevitably, excimer lasers will be able to deliver the separate hemidivisional treatment required in a single process. The reward for reduction and regularization will be better visual acuity and enhanced overall visual performance.

In recent years, the importance of the Alpins Method in studying and reporting the results of refractive surgery has become apparent.[12-16] Researchers now have a useful, comprehensive, common language in their approach to astigmatism analysis. But in terms of the sheer number of people affected, the Vector Planning approach may be the method's most significant application. Using the Vector Planning approach in patients with irregular astigmatism, every refractive surgeon can offer some level of improved care to every patient.

REFERENCES

1. Alpins NA. A new method of analyzing vectors for changes in astigmatism. *J Cataract Refract Surg.* 1993;19(4):524-533.
2. Alpins NA, Goggin M. Practical astigmatism analysis for refractive outcomes in cataract and refractive surgery. *Surv Ophthalmol.* 2004;49(1):109-122.
3. Jaffe NS, Clayman HM. *The pathophysiology of corneal astigmatism after cataract extraction. Transactions of the American Academy of Ophthalmologoy and Otolaryngology.* Rochester, MN: 1975:OP-615-OP-630.
4. Alpins NA. Treatment of irregular astigmatism. *J Cataract Refract Surg.* 1998;24(5):634-646.
5. Alpins N, Stamatelatos G. Chapter 24: The Cornea - Part X: Treatment and analysis of astigmatism during the laser era. In: Boyd BF, ed. *Modern Ophthalmology: The Highlights.* New Delhi, India: J.P. Medical Ltd; 2010:381-404.
6. Alpins NA. New method of targeting vectors to treat astigmatism. *J Cataract Refract Surg.* 1997;23(1):65-75.
7. Alpins NA. Corneal versus refractive astigmatism: integrated analysis. *Ocular Surgery News.* June 15, 1999:44.
8. Baldwin WR, Mills D. A longitudinal study of corneal astigmatism and total astigmatism. *Am J Optom Physiol Opt.* 1981;58(3):206-211.
9. Residual astigmatism and the prospective contact lens patient. 20/20 Web site. http://www.2020mag.com/ce/TTViewTest.aspx?LessonId=105459. Accessed March 28, 2014.

10. Javal E. *Memoires d'Ophthalmometrie*. Paris, France: G. Masson; 1890.

11. Goggin M, Alpins N, Schmid LM. Management of irregular astigmatism. *Curr Opin Ophthalmol.* 2000;11(4):260-266.

12. Author Information Pack. American Academy of Ophthalmology Web site. https://www.elsevier. com/wps/find/journaldescription.cws_home/620418?generatepdf=true. Accessed January 19, 2016.

13. Information for Authors. American Society of Cataract and Refractive Surgery Web site. http://www. jcrsjournal.org/content/authorinfo#info. Accessed September 1, 2016.

14. Reinstein DZ, Archer TJ, Randleman JB. JRS standard for reporting astigmatism outcomes of refractive surgery [editorial]. *J Refract Surg.* 2014;30(10):654-659.

15. Reinstein DZ, Randleman JB, Archer TJ. JRS standard for reporting outcomes of intraocular lens based refractive surgery. *J Refract Surg.* 2017;22(4):218-222.

16. Reinstein DZ, Archer TJ, Srinivasan S, et al. Standard for reporting refractive outcomes of intraocular lens-based refractive surgery. *J Cataract Refract Surg.* 2017;43(4):435-439.

Chapter 18

Polar Displays Versus Double-Angle Vector Diagrams

An Early Search for Consensus

The title of this chapter was one of the pivotal points in a fascinating email discussion among editors and invited experts representing two major ophthalmic journals—the *Journal of Refractive Surgery* (*JRS*, the journal of the International Society of Refractive Surgery, published by SLACK Incorporated) and the *Journal of Cataract & Refractive Surgery* (*JCRS*, a journal of the American Society of Cataract and Refractive Surgery [ASCRS] and the European Society of Cataract and Refractive Surgeons, published by Elsevier Incorporated). More than a dozen people participated in the exchange (see Sidebar 18-1), which comprised over 400 separate messages sent over a 2-month period (mid-October through mid-December) in 2010. The exchange brought forth many critical points that received candid and necessary attention; unfortunately, no consensus was reached at the time.

In 2014, the *JRS* published its own standard for reporting astigmatism outcomes.[1] In 2016, both the American Academy of Ophthalmology[2] (AAO) and the ASCRS[3] adopted the *JRS* standard. A consensus was finally achieved, and I believe it represents a wholly satisfactory conclusion.

Summary History of the First Six Graphs

In 1992, George O. Waring III, MD, editor of *Refractive and Corneal Surgery* (which became *JRS* in 1995), proposed a standardized format for reporting refractive surgical outcomes.[4] By 2000, a joint *JRS-JCRS* effort resulted in a set of 6 standard graphs summarizing efficacy, predictability, safety, refractive astigmatism, and stability.[5,6] Over the next decade, the graphs were refined[7] and the journal *Cornea* joined *JRS* and *JCRS* in a simultaneously published standard requiring the graphs to be used in relevant papers submitted to the journals (Figure 18-1).[8-10]

One of the 6 graphs (Figure 18-1E) is a histogram of the manifest refractive astigmatism before and after surgery. The histogram offers an immediate understanding of whether or not the astigmatic correction was successful; however, given the vectorial nature of astigmatism, a significant amount of information was not addressed. The 2014 *JRS* editorial[1] represented that journal's effort to correct this deficiency.

Alpins N. *Practical Astigmatism: Planning and Analysis* (pp 141-148).
© 2018 SLACK Incorporated.

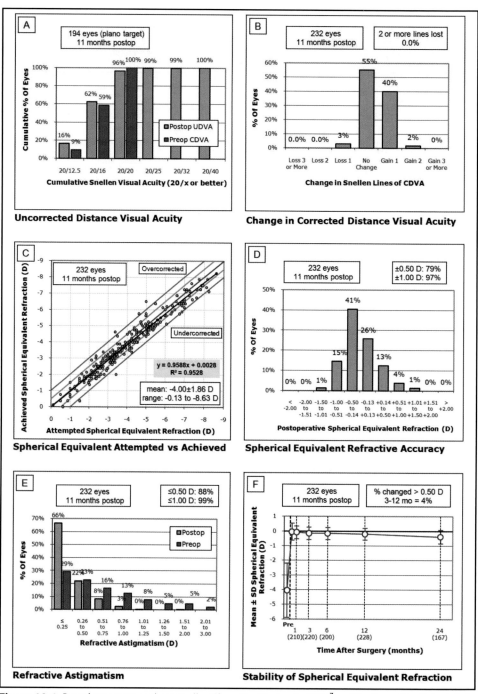

Figure 18-1. Based on a proposal originally offered by Waring in 2000[7] and furthered by Reinstein in 2009,[8] these six graphs were adopted as a reporting standard for relevant manuscripts in 2011 by JRS, JCRS, and *Cornea*.[9-11] The joint initiative indicated that the graphs "are meant to display core data that should be at the reader's fingertips for quick but meaningful comparative analysis of outcomes of essentially all refractive surgical procedures."[11] Note that graph E shows only the manifest refractive astigmatism before and after surgery, but offers no information about targeted or achieved values, nor normal astigmatism changes. (Reprinted with permission from Waring GO, III, Reinstein DZ, Dupps WJ Jr, et al. Standardized graphs and terms for refractive surgery results. *J Refract Surg*. 2011;27(1):7-9.)

Sidebar 18-1
Participants in the *JRS-JCRS* Email Exchange

More than a dozen individuals participated in an email exchange that occurred between mid-October and mid-December 2010. The group aimed to develop standardized reporting requirements for *JRS* and *JCRS*:

Ophthalmologists:
- Noel Alpins, AM, MB, BS, DO (Melb), FRANZCO, FRACS, FRCOphth, FACS
- William (BJ) Dupps Jr, MD, PhD
- Jack T. Holladay, MD
- Douglas Koch, MD
- Thomas Kohnen, MD
- Nick Mamalis, MD
- Stephen A. Obstbaum, MD
- Dan Z. Reinstein, MD, MA(Cantab), FRCOphth
- Emanuel Rosen, FRCS, FRCOphth
- R. Doyle Stulting, MD, PhD
- Li Wang, MD, PhD
- George O. Waring III, MD

Consultants:
- Timothy J. Archer, MA(Oxon), DipCompSci(Cantab)—Assistant to Dan Z. Reinstein, London Vision Clinic, London
- Professor Adrian Esterman, PhD, MSc, BSc (hons), DLSHTM—Chair of Biostatistics, Sansom Institute of Health Service Research and School of Nursing and Midwifery, University of South Australia, Adelaide
- George Stamatelatos, OD—Senior Clinical Optometrist, New Vision Clinics, Melbourne, Australia

Note—Not all participants received every email or participated in every discussion.

SETTLED TERMINOLOGY

The consensus that was eventually reached included a number of issues related to terminology. A 2006 review,[11] written by a committee of the American National Standards Institute (ANSI), altered terminology that my publications had established many years prior[12-15] and contributed to some confusion in the field[16-19] (see Foreword by Dr. Dan Z. Reinstein). The 2014 *JRS* editorial,[1] which adopts my original terminology, represents a rational endpoint both in terms of terminology and the question of polar display vs double-angle vector diagram (DAVD) in reporting astigmatism outcomes.

CLINICAL VIEW VERSUS CALCULATION

DAVDs are necessary to the performance of the vector calculations used in the Alpins Method (witness the many DAVDs in this book!). But, I have always seen DAVDs as operating in the background. They provide valuable insight for those who desire an understanding of the mathematics involved, but could be confusing, even counterproductive, for the practicing clinician. Polar plots are a more intuitive display of cylinder since clinicians are used to looking and thinking about cylinder axes from 1° to 180°. DAVDs, necessary for calculations, have no clinical value.

The following points summarize the advantages I see to polar displays over DAVDs:

- Although vector calculations are performed using DAVDs, the advantage of using polar displays is that they are much more intuitive and in step with clinical recognition of astigmatic angles as they appear on an eye compared with double-angle plots. The function of double-angle plots is to calculate from astigmatism values the clinically relevant vectors, which are then returned to polar format so they can be easily examined as they would appear on the eye, displayed at their actual axes. Revealing this double-angle mathematical process introduces unnecessary complexity.

- We are accustomed to seeing with-the-rule (WTR) astigmatism and against-the-rule (ATR) astigmatism plotted in the horizontal/vertical planes, whereas double-angle plots have WTR and ATR both on the horizontal plane. This requires clinicians to learn a different visual language for interpretation, as it does not tally with the clinical picture.

- Double-angle plots also require a readjustment in thinking—the doubled display of this mathematical (nonclinical) construct can give the incorrect perception that the axis of the vector is at double its real/true value.

- One other benefit of using a polar display is that the correction index can be plotted according to the treatment axis, so that under- or overcorrections can be seen for particular axes to highlight the presence of a systematic error at a particular axis or meridian.

MISCELLANEOUS ISSUES

Polar plots do not lend themselves to showing the familiar standard deviation ellipse. The current consensus, therefore, is to show X and Y standard deviation values in a box on single-angle polar plots.[1]

Another issue relates to the use of arithmetic vs geometric (or logarithmic) means. One argument for the use of geometric means is the following example: If two data points are 1% and 100%, what is the mean? 50.5% or 10% and why? To rephrase the question: If 2 data points are 1% (CI=0.01) and 1.99% (CI=1.99), what is the mean (D. Reinstein, T. Archer, oral communication)?

A 99% undercorrection would require changing the input value by 9900% (1/0.01 = 99.00). On the other hand, a 99% overcorrection would require changing the input value by 50% (1/1.99 = 0.502). An arithmetic mean would calculate a mean of 1—that is, the 99% overcorrection and 99% undercorrection are treated equally. A geometric mean would calculate a mean of 0.14—that is, the undercorrection is given more weight. This makes more sense because the change required to rectify the undercorrection is much greater than the change required to rectify the overcorrection.

THE NINE *JRS* STANDARD GRAPHS

The 2014 *JRS* standard[1] presents the 9 graphs shown in Figure 18-2. The 2 graphs in the lower right (Figures 18-2G and 18-2H) depict astigmatic treatments. The value of these graphs should be immediately apparent. Figure 18-2G (surgically induced astigmatism vector vs target induced astigmatism vector) answers 2 questions:

1. Did the attempted astigmatic treatment magnitude undercorrect or overcorrect?
2. Did the under/overcorrection depend on the magnitude of treatment?

Figure 18-2H answers the question: Was there a consistent rotational error? That is, was the applied treatment axis consistently clockwise or counterclockwise to the intended treatment axis?

The 2014 *JRS* standard[1] also recommends the four polar displays shown in Figure 18-3. These graphs are based on the Alpins Method and are suggested for studies in which astigmatism correction is central, or where there is a particularly interesting outcome related to astigmatism. Again, the 9 standard graphs are basic, but the journal welcomes authors to go beyond the basics if doing so will elucidate additional relevant information. The Alpins Method is recommended for those who wish to go above and beyond in reporting astigmatism outcomes.

The 2014 *JRS* editorial[1] is a good read and represents the basis for the astigmatism reporting standards used now in the peer-reviewed literature. I congratulate the *JRS* for moving the field ahead in this manner.

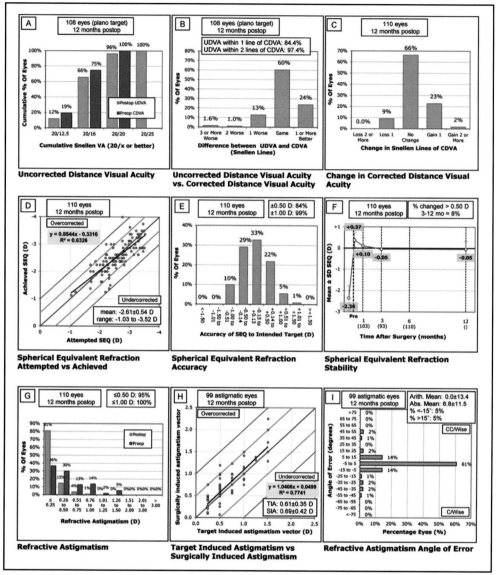

Figure 18-2. *JRS* added 2 new graphs, G and H—on astigmatism outcomes—to the 6 graphs used as a reporting standard by *JRS*, the *JCRS*, and the journal *Cornea*.[8-11] A histogram on visual acuity (B) also was added, showing the difference (in Snellen lines) between postoperative uncorrected distance visual acuity (UDVA) and preoperative correct distance visual acuity (CDVA). Abbreviation: SEQ, spherical equivalent refraction. (Reprinted with permission from Reinstein DZ, Archer TJ, Randleman JB. JRS standard for reporting astigmatism outcomes of refractive surgery [editorial]. *J Refract Surg.* 2014;30(10):654-659.)

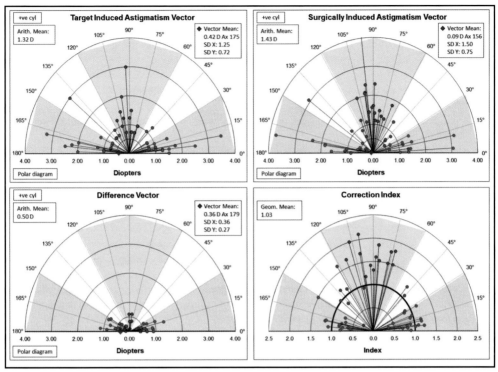

Figure 18-3. *JRS* recommended using these single-angle polar plots, based on the Alpins Method, to report outcomes for astigmatism correction in relevant studies.[1] The vector means are plotted as a red diamond (calculated using double-angle vectors, not shown) and the standard deviations for the X and Y directions are boxed in each graph. Abbreviations: CI, correction index; DV, difference vector; SIA, surgically induced astigmatism vector; TIA, target induced astigmatism vector. (Reprinted with permission from Reinstein DZ, Archer TJ, Randleman JB. JRS standard for reporting astigmatism outcomes of refractive surgery [editorial]. *J Refract Surg.* 2014;30(10):654-659.)

REFERENCES

1. Reinstein DZ, Archer TJ, Randleman JB. JRS standard for reporting astigmatism outcomes of refractive surgery [editorial]. *J Refract Surg.* 2014;30(10):654-659.
2. Author Information Pack. American Academy of Ophthalmology Web site. https://www.elsevier.com/wps/find/journaldescription.cws_home/620418?generatepdf=true. Accessed January 19, 2016.
3. Information for Authors. American Society of Cataract and Refractive Surgery Web site. http://www.jcrsjournal.org/content/authorinfo#info. Accessed September 1, 2016.
4. Waring GOI. Standardized data collection and reporting for refractive surgery. *Refract Corneal Surg.* 1992;8(suppl):1-42.
5. Koch DD, Kohnen T, Obstbaum SA, Rosen ES. Format for reporting refractive surgical data. *J Cataract Refract Surg.* 1998;24(3):285-287.
6. Waring GO, III. Standard graphs for reporting refractive surgery. *J Refract Surg.* 2000;16(4):459-466.
7. Reinstein DZ, Waring GO, III. Graphic reporting of outcomes of refractive surgery. *J Refract Surg.* 2009;25(11):975-978.
8. Dupps WJ, Jr., Kohnen T, Mamalis N, et al. Standardized graphs and terms for refractive surgery results. *J Cataract Refract Surg.* 2011;37(1):1-3.
9. Stulting RD, Dupps WJ, Jr., Kohnen T, et al. Standardized graphs and terms for refractive surgery results. *Cornea.* 2011;30(8):945-947.

10. Waring GO, III, Reinstein DZ, Dupps WJ Jr, et al. Standardized graphs and terms for refractive surgery results. *J Refract Surg.* 2011;27(1):7-9.

11. Eydelman MB, Drum B, Holladay J, et al. Standardized analyses of correction of astigmatism by laser systems that reshape the cornea. *J Refract Surg.* 2006;22(1):81-95.

12. Alpins N. Terms used for the analysis of astigmatism [letter]. *J Refract Surg.* 2006;22(6):528-529.

13. Alpins NA. A new method of analyzing vectors for changes in astigmatism. *J Cataract Refract Surg.* 1993;19(4):524-33.

14. Alpins NA. New method of targeting vectors to treat astigmatism. *J Cataract Refract Surg.* 1997;23(1):65-75.

15. Alpins NA. Vector analysis of astigmatism changes by flattening, steepening, and torque. *J Cataract Refract Surg.* 1997;23(10):1503-1514.

16. Alpins N. Astigmatism terminology and source references [letter]. *J Cataract Refract Surg.* 2016;42(4):643.

17. St Clair RM, Sharma A, Huang D, et al. Development of a nomogram for femtosecond laser astigmatic keratotomy for astigmatism after keratoplasty. *J Cataract Refract Surg.* 2016;42(4):556-562.

18. Trivizki O, Levinger E, Levinger S. Correction ratio and vector analysis of femtosecond laser arcuate keratotomy for the correction of post-mushroom profile keratoplasty astigmatism. *J Cataract Refract Surg.* 2015;41(9):1973-1979.

19. Schallhorn S, Brown M, Venter J, Teenan D, Hettinger K, Yamamoto H. Early clinical outcomes of wavefront-guided myopic LASIK treatments using a new-generation Hartmann-Shack aberrometer. *J Refract Surg.* 2014;30(1):14-21.

Chapter 19

Clinical Application of the Alpins Method for Clinical Studies

A CLINICAL TOOL WELL-STUDIED

The basic mathematics and terminology of the Alpins Method were spelled out primarily in four papers between 1993 and 2001.[1-4] As shown in Table 19-1, these papers have been cited many times. Not included in the table are many other papers, letters, editorials, book chapters, interviews, etc, that I have published throughout the years with or without coauthors.

As described in Chapter 20, a group from the American National Standards Institute (ANSI) promulgated obfuscatory terminology[5] that may have been cited more than 40 times in the literature, often necessitating remedial action by myself or others.[6-13] To those others, I give sincere thanks. Fortunately, I think the collateral damage will subside in time. The episode is described in greater detail in Chapter 20.

Perhaps the most satisfying use of the Alpins Method, to my way of thinking, is not to verify, refute, confirm, supplement, amend, or append the method itself in any way, but simply to use it as the tool it is meant to be—as a means to analyze or compare astigmatic outcomes for individual patients or groups of patients, or to assess the accuracy of equipment or the predictability of surgical approaches that correct astigmatism. After all, a tool can hardly have a clinical application if it is not clinically useful.

A FAN OF FAN GRAPHS

The Alpins Method has been used in many studies in conjunction with many different types of surgery, listed here in no particular order:

- Incisional refractive surgery[14,15]
- Laser refractive surgery[16-25]
- Arcuate incisions[23]
- Collagen crosslinking in keratoconic corneas previously treated with intracorneal ring segments[26]
- Orthokeratology[27]

Alpins N. *Practical Astigmatism:*
Planning and Analysis (pp 149-156).
© 2018 SLACK Incorporated.

		Table19-1	
		Signature Publications of the Alpins Method (Number of Citations Per ResearchGate, Accessed 12 October 2016)	
Year	**Journal**	**Title**	**Number of Citations**
1993	*J Cataract Refract Surg*	A new method of analyzing vectors for changes in astigmatism[2]	241
1997	*J Cataract Refract Surg*	New method of targeting vectors to treat astigmatism[3]	114
1997	*J Cataract Refract Surg*	Vector analysis of astigmatism changes by flattening, steepening, and torque[4]	101
2001	*J Cataract Refract Surg*	Astigmatism analysis by the Alpins method[1]	202

- Cataract/intraocular lens (IOL) surgery[28-30]
- Vitrectomy[31]
- Higher-order aberrations [32]

One thread common to many of these studies is the use of single-angle plots, or "fan graphs," as they are sometimes called. The editors of the *Journal of Refractive Surgery* (*JRS*) came down in favor of single-angle plots in their standard for astigmatism reporting published in 2014.[33] It would be 2 years before *Journal of Cataract & Refractive Surgery* and the journal *Ophthalmology* would follow suit.[34,35]

Single-angle plots have the simple advantage of coinciding with the clinician's intuitive understanding of astigmatic meridia on the cornea. The relative advantages and disadvantages of single-angle vs double-angle plots, as well as examples of the single-angle plots used in the *JRS* astigmatism-reporting standard, are further described in Chapter 18.

An excellent example of single-angle plots at work is shown in Figure 19-1, from an article by Archer et al[24] published in 2015 by *JRS*. The article confirmed that ocular residual astigmatism (ORA) in "normal" patients can be more than 1.25 D, and the predictability of refractive cylinder correction is lower in patients with high ORA (although the difference appeared to be lower than in previous reports, as the amount of cylinder treated was not matched between patient groups in these studies). Eyes most at risk for a less accurate astigmatic outcome in this study were those with high ORA and high corneal astigmatism.

I was an early advocate of fan graphs precisely for the reason noted above—that they were intuitively understandable by the clinician. However, I would point out that they are not vector diagrams; they simply show—immediately and obviously—the axis

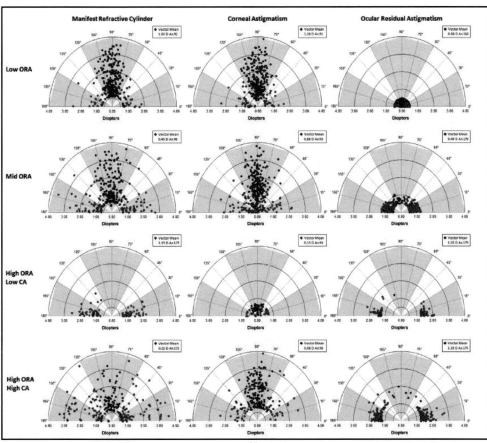

Figure 19-1. In a retrospective study, Archer et al[24] used polar plots to differentiate between low-, mid-, and high-ORA groups, and also between low and high corneal astigmatism in the high-ORA group. Matching for the manifest refractive cylinder (MRC) and grouping by ORA magnitude resulted in similar predictability; however, eyes with high ORA and high corneal astigmatism were less predictable. Abbreviations: Ax, axis; CA, corneal astigmatism; ORA, ocular residual astigmatism. (Reprinted from *Journal of Cataract & Refractive Surgery,* 41/7, Archer TJ, Reinstein DZ, Pinero DP, Gobbe M, Carp GI, Comparison of the predictability of refractive cylinder correction by laser in situ keratomileusis in eyes with low or high ocular residual astigmatism, 10, Copyright 2015, with permission from Elsevier.)

of the vector as it would appear on an eye; and the relative length of the coordinate lines provides a visual guide to the amount of astigmatism at the meridian indicated. From my early work with double-angle vector diagrams[2], which are used "behind the scenes" to calculate the various indices of the Alpins Method, I simply halved the axes in order to show where the astigmatism or the vectorial change would be found on the cornea given the clinician's typical vantage point. To me, the single-angle plot compared with the double-angle plot was simply more clinically useful.

EXAMPLES OF THE ALPINS METHOD IN CLINICAL STUDIES

As shown in Table 19-2, clinical studies utilizing the Alpins Method run the gamut of subject matter.

Table 19-2		
Clinical Studies Utilizing the Alpins Method in the Peer-Reviewed Literature		
Authors, Year	**Title**	**How the Alpins Method Was Used**
Plech AR et al, 2010[32]	Corneal higher-order aberrations in amblyopia	ORA was calculated as the vectorial difference between refractive and corneal astigmatism, and shown in single-angle plots and double-angle vector diagrams
Alio JL et al, 2010[29]	Microincision cataract surgery with toric IOL implantation for correcting moderate and high astigmatism: pilot study	Vector analysis was done by the Alpins Method; standard terminology (TIA, SIA, etc.) and indices (correction index, magnitude of error, angle of error, etc) were used; vectorial display of TIAs with summated mean was shown in single-angle plot
Bucher C et al, 2010[22]	Corneal limbal marking in the treatment of myopic astigmatism with the excimer laser	Refractive and topographic data were analyzed using vector analysis; standard terminology (SIA, TIA, etc) and indices (angle of error, difference vector) were used
Pinero DP et al, 2010[36]	Modification and refinement of astigmatism in keratoconic eyes with intrastromal corneal ring segments	Alpins vector analysis was performed using AS-SORT software; standard terminology (SIA, TIA, DV, etc) and indices (magnitude of error, angle of error, FE, etc) were used
Alio JL et al, 2011[30]	Vector analysis of astigmatic changes after cataract surgery with implantation of a new toric multifocal IOL	Vector analysis (magnitude and orientation) was used after implantation of 2 toric IOL models; standard terminology and indices were used; vectorial display of the DV during the postoperative follow-up was shown in single-angle plot

(continued)

The Alpins Method lends itself to any ocular procedure where corneal and refractive astigmatism are variables that ought to be assessed preoperatively and postoperatively—which pretty much covers every ocular procedure in a seeing eye. As noted, the terminology and indices defined by the method constitute a common language and allow for statistical uniformity across the vast spectrum of conditions treated by the modern ophthalmologist. It is perhaps a vital test of a widely used ophthalmic technique that meaningful information can be shared by those whose interests extend to cataract surgery, toric intraocular lenses (IOLs), incisional keratotomy, keratoconus, collagen cross-linking, intracorneal ring segments, and/or the pervasive variety of laser refractive surgical techniques existent today.

Table19-2 (continued)
Clinical Studies Utilizing the Alpins Method in the Peer-Reviewed Literature

Authors, Year	Title	How the Alpins Method Was Used
Pinero DP et al, 2012[26]	Vectorial astigmatic changes after corneal collagen crosslinking in keratoconic corneas previously treated with intracorneal ring segments: a preliminary study	Calculations were performed using the ASSORT software; standard terminology (TIA, SIA, DV, etc) and indices (ME, AE, FE, TRQ, etc) were used; vectorial display of DV during postoperative follow-up was shown in single-angle plot
Ruckl T et al, 2013[23]	Femtosecond laser-assisted intrastromal arcuate keratotomy to reduce corneal astigmatism	Vector analysis and graphic displays were performed using the Alpins Method and ASSORT program; standard terminology (TIA, SIA, DV, etc) and indices (correction index) were used and graphed as single-angle plots
Qian Y et al, 2015[25]	Influence of intraocular astigmatism on the correction of myopic astigmatism by femtosecond laser small-incision lenticule extraction	ORA was determined by vector analysis using manifest refraction and Scheimpflug camera imaging of the anterior cornea; SIA in high- and low-ORA patients was shown in single-angle plots

Abbreviations: DV, difference vector; FE, flattening effect; IOL, intraocular lens; ORA, ocular residual astigmatism; SIA, surgically induced astigmatism vector; TIA, target induced astigmatism vector; TRQ, torque.

AND THIS IS IMPORTANT BECAUSE?

It is gratifying that the Alpins Method has proved to be a valuable tool to the hundreds of investigators who have worked so hard and risked so much to design, implement, and publish the clinical studies that have been cited in this chapter—not to mention the thousands of courageous patients who consciously entrusted these researchers with their health and welfare. Although I had great confidence in my methodology from the very beginning, it is truly humbling for these events to have unfolded in a field populated by huge intellects and world-renowned personages—a field to which I have devoted my career, and which I chose at an age that I now think of as rather young and tender. I consider myself extremely lucky, and forever indebted to many colleagues, teachers, and mentors, most of whom I hope I have mentioned herein at least in passing.

I'll take this opportunity to thank a few colleagues not mentioned elsewhere in this book (again, in no particular order): Michael Goggin, who has written letters to journal editors correcting the misuse of the terminology I introduced, and has presented with me, most years for the past 20 years, at my course on astigmatism treatment and analysis at the annual meetings of the American Society of Cataract and Refractive Surgery and the European Society of Cataract and Refractive Surgeons; Ming X. Wang, who quickly understood the value of the Vector Planning approach and invited me to write chapters in several books, and Lance Kugler, who in 2010 coauthored with Dr. Wang an important paper on patients with high ORA; Bruce Wallace, who oversaw a surgical techniques column in *Ocular Surgery News* in the 1990s; Jorge Alio, who has used the Alpins Method in multiple publications and coauthored an editorial on terminology with me; Günther Grabner, of Salzburg, Austria, who published articles using the Alpins Method; J. Bradley Randleman, a coauthor of the 2014 *JRS* astigmatism reporting standard; Maria Clara Arbelaez and Samuel Arba-Mosquera, who have worked with me and reported results using the Alpins Method; and Sandra Belmont and Kurt Buzard, who invited me to teach courses at the annual meetings of the American Society of Cataract and Refractive Surgery in the early 1990s.

I also owe thanks to many non-ophthalmologists: Doug Mastel, of Mastel Precision, who early on became a supporter of the ASSORT (Alpins Statistical System for Ophthalmic Refractive surgery Techniques) program and the Alpins Method, displaying the program in his booth at professional meetings; Renzo Mattioli headed the efforts to incorporate iASSORT into the Keratron Scout corneal topographer; James Ong is a mathematics wizard who helped me with many initiatives and publications; David P. Piñero, of Alicante, Spain, is an optometrist and editor of an optometry journal, who has taught many courses with me and published studies of ORA; and many others whom I have tried to mention throughout this book.

This support is extremely gratifying to me. Another source of supreme satisfaction is the way individual practitioners are using the method, as programmed into various available software and calculators (see Chapter 24), to refine their results over time and provide better visual outcomes for their patients. Consistent use of these tools brings into stark relief recurring over- or undercorrections, or off-axis treatments predictably clockwise or counterclockwise to their desired location—and for toric IOL implantation as well as for refractive laser correction. I receive many reports from individual surgeons who alter their nomograms or adjust their equipment after identifying the type of errors described. The software programs described in Chapter 24 provide a dependable roadmap to this kind of improved surgical outcome, which I hope will extend to every reader of this text.

REFERENCES

1. Alpins N. Astigmatism analysis by the Alpins method. *J Cataract Refract Surg.* 2001;27(1):31-49.
2. Alpins NA. A new method of analyzing vectors for changes in astigmatism. *J Cataract Refract Surg.* 1993;19(4):524-533.
3. Alpins NA. New method of targeting vectors to treat astigmatism. *J Cataract Refract Surg.* 1997;23(1):65-75.
4. Alpins NA. Vector analysis of astigmatism changes by flattening, steepening, and torque. *J Cataract Refract Surg.* 1997;23(10):1503-1514.
5. Eydelman MB, Drum B, Holladay J, et al. Standardized analyses of correction of astigmatism by laser systems that reshape the cornea. *J Refract Surg.* 2006;22(1):81-95.

6. Alpins N. Terms used for the analysis of astigmatism [letter]. *J Refract Surg.* 2006;22(6):528-529.

7. Masket S. Special articles and peer review [letter]. *J Refract Surg.* 2007;23(2):115.

8. Goggin M. More on astigmatism analysis [letter]. *J Refract Surg.* 2007;23(5):430-431.

9. Alio JL, Alpins N. Excimer laser correction of astigmatism: consistent terminology for better outcomes. *J Refract Surg.* 201;30(5):4294-4295.

10. Alpins N. Vector analysis with the femtosecond laser [letter]. *J Cataract Refract Surg.* 2014;40(7):1246-1247.

11. Pinero DP. Terminology and referencing of astigmatic vector analysis [letter]. *J Cataract Refract Surg.* 2013;39(11):1792.

12. Dupps WJ, Jr. Impact of citation practices: beyond journal impact factors [editorial]. *J Cataract Refract Surg.* 2008;34(9):1419-1421.

13. Alpins N. Astigmatism terminology and source references [letter]. *J Cataract Refract Surg.* 2016;42(4):643.

14. Hoffart L, Proust H, Matonti F, Conrath J, Ridings B. Correction of postkeratoplasty astigmatism by femtosecond laser compared with mechanized astigmatic keratotomy. *Am J Ophthalmol.* 2009;147(5):779-787

15. Wang L, Misra M, Koch DD. Peripheral corneal relaxing incisions combined with cataract surgery. *J Cataract Refract Surg.* 2003;29(4):712-722.

16. Alpins N, Stamatelatos G. Clinical outcomes of laser in situ keratomileusis using combined topography and refractive wavefront treatments for myopic astigmatism. *J Cataract Refract Surg.* 2008;34(8):1250-1259.

17. Gan D, Zhou X, Dai J et al. Outcomes of epi-LASIK for the correction of high myopia and myopic astigmatism after more than 1 year. *Ophthalmologica.* 2009;223(2):102-110.

18. Alpins NA, Taylor HR, Kent DG, et al. Three multizone photorefractive keratectomy algorithms for myopia. The Melbourne Excimer Laser Group. *J Refract Surg.* 1997;13(6):535-544.

19. Febbraro JL, ron-Rosa D, Gross M, Aron B, Bremond-Gignac D. One year clinical results of photoastigmatic refractive keratectomy for compound myopic astigmatism. *J Cataract Refract Surg.* 1999;25(7):911-920.

20. Taylor HR, Guest CS, Kelly P, Alpins NA. Comparison of excimer laser treatment of astigmatism and myopia. The Excimer Laser and Research Group. *Arch Ophthalmol.* 1993;111(12):1621-1626.

21. Taylor HR, Kelly P, Alpins N. Excimer laser correction of myopic astigmatism. *J Cataract Refract Surg.* 1994;20 Suppl:243-251.

22. Bucher C, Zuberbuhler B, Goggin M, Esterman A, Schipper I. Corneal limbal marking in the treatment of myopic astigmatism with the excimer laser. *J Refract Surg.* 2010;26(7):505-511.

23. Ruckl T, Dexl AK, Bachernegg A, et al. Femtosecond laser-assisted intrastromal arcuate keratotomy to reduce corneal astigmatism. *J Cataract Refract Surg.* 2013;39(4):528-538.

24. Archer TJ, Reinstein DZ, Pinero DP, Gobbe M, Carp GI. Comparison of the predictability of refractive cylinder correction by laser in situ keratomileusis in eyes with low or high ocular residual astigmatism. *J Cataract Refract Surg.* 2015;41(7):1383-1392.

25. Qian Y, Huang J, Chu R, et al. Influence of intraocular astigmatism on the correction of myopic astigmatism by femtosecond laser small-incision lenticule extraction. *J Cataract Refract Surg.* 2015;41(5):1057-1064.

26. Pinero DP, Alio JL, Klonowski P, Toffaha B. Vectorial astigmatic changes after corneal collagen crosslinking in keratoconic corneas previously treated with intracorneal ring segments: a preliminary study. *Eur J Ophthalmol.* 2012;22Suppl7:S69-S80.

27. Mountford J, Pesudovs K. An analysis of the astigmatic changes induced by accelerated orthokeratology. *Clin Exp Optom.* 2002;85(5):284-293.

28. Morcillo-Laiz R, Zato MA, Munoz-Negrete FJ, rnalich-Montiel F. Surgically induced astigmatism after biaxial phacoemulsification compared to coaxial phacoemulsification. *Eye (Lond).* 2009;23(4):835-839.

29. Alio JL, Agdeppa MC, Pongo VC, El KB. Microincision cataract surgery with toric intraocular lens implantation for correcting moderate and high astigmatism: pilot study. *J Cataract Refract Surg.* 2010;36(1):44-52.

30. Alio JL, Pinero DP, Tomas J, Plaza AB. Vector analysis of astigmatic changes after cataract surgery with implantation of a new toric multifocal intraocular lens. *J Cataract Refract Surg.* 2011;37(7):1217-1229.

31. Galway G, Drury B, Cronin BG, Bourke RD. A comparison of induced astigmatism in 20- vs 25-gauge vitrectomy procedures. *Eye (Lond).* 2010;24(2):315-317.

32. Plech AR, Pinero DP, Laria C, Aleson A, Alio JL. Corneal higher-order aberrations in amblyopia. *Eur J Ophthalmol.* 2010;20(1):12-20.

33. Reinstein DZ, Archer TJ, Randleman JB. JRS standard for reporting astigmatism outcomes of refractive surgery [editorial]. *J Refract Surg.* 2014;30(10):654-659.

34. Author Information Pack. American Academy of Ophthalmology Web site. https://www.elsevier.com/wps/find/journaldescription.cws_home/620418?generatepdf=true. Accessed January 19, 2016.

35. Information for Authors. American Society of Cataract and Refractive Surgery Web site. http://www.jcrsjournal.org/content/authorinfo#info. Accessed September 1, 2016.

36. Pinero DP, Alio JL, Teus MA, Barraquer RI, Michael R, Jimenez R. Modification and refinement of astigmatism in keratoconic eyes with intrastromal corneal ring segments. *J Cataract Refract Surg.* 2010;36(9):1562-1572.

Chapter 20

Regulatory Adoption

THE CASE OF THE RUNAWAY PROJECT GROUP

The influence of the US Food and Drug Administration (FDA) on cataract and refractive surgery is substantial. As a result, if this locomotive of a regulatory agency ever jumps the track, any number of companies, researchers, and individual practitioners can be severely dented.

My case is an excellent example. It will take some explaining, but like a train wreck, it is difficult to look away.

As with many governmental initiatives, even the titles of the participating organizations can be ponderous. In 2006, a paper was published in the *Journal of Refractive Surgery* (*JRS*), written by Eydelman et al.[1] The authors represented an "Astigmatism Project group…created under the auspices of the American National Standards Institute (ANSI) Z80.11 Working Group on Laser Systems for Corneal Reshaping." So, they comprised a project group as a working group of ANSI (which is a 501[c]3 private, not-for-profit organization founded in 1918[2]). The field would discover later[3-5] that the paper was not subjected to peer review, but in deference to acknowledging its respected source, was published as submitted without acknowledging the original source and terminology, a fact I find surprising. In response to one complaint that the lack of peer review should have at least been disclosed,[4] the editor of *JRS* at the time, George O. Waring, III, MD, acknowledged that "articles that have not undergone peer review should be labeled as such." But Dr. Waring continued to hold that it would have been "inappropriate" to submit the ANSI report to peer review.

Two years prior to publication of the ANSI paper—in November 2004—the lead author, Malvina Eydelman, introduced herself to the field in an article she wrote for *EyeWorld*, titled "FDA's Role in the Ophthalmic Device Evaluation Process."[6] She wrote that she was an ophthalmologist and "medical officer in the US Food and Drug Administration Center for Devices and Radiological Health/Division of Ophthalmic and ENT Devices." At this writing, Eydelman is quoted in the Wikipedia entry for laser in situ keratomileusis (LASIK), which cites a presentation she gave at the October 2014 annual meeting of the American Academy of Ophthalmology (AAO).[7] An article pub-

Alpins N. *Practical Astigmatism:
Planning and Analysis* (pp 157-163).
© 2018 SLACK Incorporated.

lished on the *EyeWorld* website in November 2011, titled "Innovation in Ophthalmology: Walking the FDA Tightrope,"[8] identified Dr. Eydelman as director of the FDA's Division of Ophthalmic and ENT Devices, Center for Devices and Radiological Health.

I describe Dr. Eydelman's FDA position carefully only because it is estimable, carrying with it significant influence and responsibility. Her coauthors on the 2006 ANSI paper, in the order in which they are listed, were Bruce Drum, PhD; Jack Holladay, MD, MSEE, FACS; Gene Hilmantel, OD, MS; Guy Kezirian, MD; Daniel Durrie, MD; R. Doyle Stulting, MD, PhD; Donald Sanders, MD, PhD; and Bonita Wong, OD, MSc.[1] In March 2009, the FDA officially recognized the ANSI paper as a standard for the performance of LASIK.[9]

In reality, this project group as the working group of the private, not-for-profit standards organization in my opinion had jumped the rails, without proper acknowledgement of the source and original astigmatic terminology, and the group's non-peer-reviewed paper would continue to obfuscate ophthalmology terminology for years to come. For more than a decade, many people in the field worked to repair the damage, but terminology errors continued to emerge in the ophthalmic literature like the relentless critters in the carnival whack-a-mole game.

RESCUE EFFORTS *AD INFINITUM*

The terminology that I described in 1993[10], 1997,[11,12] and 2001[13] was adopted relatively recently as a reporting standard by three major ophthalmic publications, *JRS*[14], the *Journal of Cataract & Refractive Surgery (JCRS)*,[15] and *Ophthalmology*,[16] the journal of the AAO. In their guidance to authors, the *JCRS*, the official journal of the American Society of Cataract and Refractive Surgery and the European Society of Cataract and Refractive Surgeons, and the AAO, simply accepted what had been spelled out by *JRS* in 2014.

As described in Chapter 19, many clinical studies have employed the Alpins Method in reporting the results of incisional refractive surgery,[17,18] laser refractive surgery,[19-24] cataract/intraocular lens surgery,[25-27] vitrectomy,[28] and orthokeratology.[29] Unfortunately, many other studies have misused or ignored the terminology that was established in my early publications.[10,11,13] Many authors, including myself, have attempted to correct these errors when they occurred.[3-5,30-34] Yet, the erroneous terms introduced by the ANSI authors (Table 20-1) can be found in scores of papers. In fact, the careening trajectory of the ANSI project group, I think, was a significant hindrance to scientific ophthalmology and the sincere efforts of hundreds of researchers and thousands of practitioners around the world. Terminology errors continue to crop up, even in *JCRS*.[35-38]

There were a number of heroic efforts to restore order in the wake of the original 2006 ANSI paper; central among them, in my opinion, was an editorial by William BJ. Dupps, Jr, MD, PhD, published in 2008 in *JCRS*.[33] Dr. Dupps did an amazing job of describing the many ways that peer-reviewed publishing can be distorted or misleading, and how to avoid those mistakes.

Table 20-1
Incorrect ANSI Terminology Versus Accepted Alpins Method Terminology

Incorrect Terminology	Correct Terminology
Eydelman et al[1] (2006)	*Alpins Method[10-16] (1993, 1997, 2001, 2014, 2016)*
Intended refractive correction (IRC)	Target induced astigmatism vector (TIA)
Surgically induced refractive correction (SIRC)	Surgically induced astigmatism vector (SIA)
Error of magnitude	Magnitude of error
Error of angle	Angle of error
Error vector	Difference vector (DV)
Error ratio	Index of success
Correction ratio	Correction index

Abbreviation: ANSI, American National Standards Institute.

Dr. Dupps referred specifically to my work in the following passage[33]:

Finally, omission of key references or attribution of work to a secondary reference rather than a primary source can distort the field by re-mapping key contributions inaccurately. This challenging issue, a recently noted example of which is Alpins'[10] under-acknowledged vector approach to analyzing surgically induced astigmatism, can be addressed through errata and correspondences[39]; but once in the literature, such errors are prone to propagation. Errors of omission or inaccurate attribution also occur when review articles are used in lieu of primary sources.

Here is an example of how deficient referencing can lead to claims of novelty in the face of previously described and widely accepted techniques. A recent paper by Kanellopoulos[40] on "topography-modified refraction...in myopic topography-guided LASIK" described the use of topographic and refractive parameters in developing a treatment plan, making no reference to my previous work on the topic.[11,19,42,43] Although the issue was raised soon after publication of the web-based paper[41], the author declined to provide complete referencing, which opens the door to ongoing fallacious claims of novelty.

It is worth noting that Dr. Dupps' instructional editorial[33] was published in 2008, only two years after the 2006 ANSI review. It would take another 6 years after Dr. Dupps' editorial in 2014 for *JRS* to publish its own standards,[14] which incorporate all elements of the Alpins Method, and 8 years for the *JCRS*[15] and *Ophthalmology*[16] to recommend the Alpins Method to authors for reporting astigmatism outcomes.

Terminology Inconsistencies in *JCRS*

Dr. Douglas Koch of the *JCRS* has lauded the Alpins Method in a number of publications between 1997 and 2006.[39,44-46] He called the Alpins Method "one of the more sophisticated approaches"[44] and cited its "elegance and usefulness."[39] After I responded to the terminology errors made in a 2013 *JCRS* paper by Kunert et al,[35] my letter to the editor[31] was followed by this editors' note:

> We agree: It is important to recognize and reference Alpins[10] pioneering work in this area and particularly the analytical system that he developed, a modified version of which was described by Eydelman et al[1]. For purposes of clarity and consistency with the majority of papers that use this type of analysis, we recommend that authors use Alpins[10] original terms and equations.

The *JCRS* editors apparently did not follow their own advice, as evidenced by the terminology errors in a 2015 *JCRS* paper by Trivizki et al.[37] I responded to this paper with a letter[34] that was published in the same issue of *JCRS* as another paper[36] with erroneous terminology. I described these errors to Dr. Dupps in an email, and the *JCRS* author guidelines[15] were modified shortly thereafter. So, I am hopeful that the use and citation of the flawed ANSI terminology in the literature will trickle to a stop.

Whatever the reason for the terminology inconsistencies, it is gratifying to see that, in 2016, Dr. Dupps and the editorial team at *JCRS* have recommended my method to authors when reporting astigmatism outcomes.[15]

Response to Publication of the *JRS* Standard

In contrast, the publication by *JRS* of a new standard for astigmatism reporting[14] sets the highest example for scientific publishing. It was a significant and commendable accomplishment.

A small note of dissatisfaction, perhaps, came in the form of a letter from Kristian Næser, of Denmark.[43] Responding to the publication of the *JRS* standard, Dr. Naeser suggested some revisions both in terminology and graphic presentation. Dr. Naeser's full letter and the response from *JRS* editors Dan Z. Reinstein and Timothy J. Archer, of London, are well worth a read. Suffice it here for me to say that, what the ANSI paper did to my previously described terminology, Dr. Naeser attempted to do with the concepts I introduced in my paper on flattening, steepening, and torque.[12] Here is an excerpt from the *JRS* editors' response to Dr. Naeser[47]:

> The vector calculations described in Dr. Næser's example are identical to those described by the Alpins method, except that Dr. Næser's calculations have normalized the vectors with reference to the surgical meridian. However, the

terminology is somewhat different to that described by Alpins; for example, Dr. Næser's term "error in astigmatism" is equivalent to the Alpins term "difference vector." This is an example of the confusion that is introduced for the non-astigmatism expert when reading different articles reporting astigmatism outcomes. Our goal was to provide consistency of terminology for the reader given that the mathematics of the majority of vector analysis methods are essentially identical.

The editors go on to say that the *JRS* standard was not meant to cover all studies, and that authors are encouraged to submit more complex analyses, etc. A more detailed description of the *JRS* standard can be found in Chapter 18, including the basic graphs and single-angle polar plots that should be used, where appropriate.

The title of this chapter, "Regulatory Adoption," is, perhaps, both a little sarcastic and a little wishful. It is sarcastic in that the "official" FDA position[9] when it comes to analyzing the safety and efficacy of the very expensive instrumentation surrounding refractive surgery—the lasers and corneal measurement devices subject to FDA oversight—apparently still holds to the 2006 ANSI paper. It is wishful in that the standards of peer-reviewed, scientific ophthalmic publishing, which have widely adopted the Alpins Method, apparently remain unacknowledged by a major American medical regulatory agency; and we wish that were not the case. We hope that science and academic standards could lead governmental regulations and not the other way around.

The obvious solution is for Eydelman et al[1], the original authors of the 2006 ANSI paper, to petition the FDA to amend the agency's 2009 adoption of the ANSI paper as a standard for reporting LASIK results, or to correct the flawed terminology. In this way, the FDA will demonstrate its determination to allow experts in the field to create and promulgate accepted standards.

References

1. Eydelman MB, Drum B, Holladay J, et al. Standardized analyses of correction of astigmatism by laser systems that reshape the cornea. *J Refract Surg*. 2006;22(1):81-95.
2. About ANSI. American National Standards Institute Web site. http://www.ansi.org/about_ansi/overview/overview.aspx?menuid=1. Accessed January 18, 2016.
3. Alpins N. Terms used for the analysis of astigmatism [letter]. *J Refract Surg*. 2006;22(6):528-529.
4. Masket S. Special articles and peer review [letter]. *J Refract Surg*. 2007;23(2):115.
5. Goggin M. More on astigmatism analysis [letter]. *J Refract Surg*. 2007;23(5):430-431.
6. Eydelman M. FDA's role in the ophthalmic device evaluation process. EyeWorld Web site. http://www.eyeworld.org/article.php?sid=2082.
7. LASIK. Wikipedia Web site. https://en.wikipedia.org/wiki/LASIK.
8. Lipner M. Innovation in ophthalmology: walking the FDA tightrope. EyeWorld Web site. http://www.eyeworld.org/article.php?sid=6113.
9. Latest on FDA's LASIK program: FDA recognition of ANSI laser systems for corneal reshaping. FDA Web site. http://www.fda.gov/MedicalDevices/ProductsandMedicalProcedures/SurgeryandLifeSupport/LASIK/ucm061421.htm. Accessed January 18, 2016.
10. Alpins NA. A new method of analyzing vectors for changes in astigmatism. *J Cataract Refract Surg*. 1993;19(4):524-533.
11. Alpins NA. New method of targeting vectors to treat astigmatism. *J Cataract Refract Surg*. 1997;23(1):65-75.

12. Alpins NA. Vector analysis of astigmatism changes by flattening, steepening, and torque. *J Cataract Refract Surg.* 1997;23(10):1503-1514.

13. Alpins N. Astigmatism analysis by the Alpins method. *J Cataract Refract Surg.* 2001;27(1):31-49.

14. Reinstein DZ, Archer TJ, Randleman JB. JRS standard for reporting astigmatism outcomes of refractive surgery [editorial]. *J Refract Surg.* 2014;30(10):654-659.

15. Information for Authors. American Society of Cataract and Refractive Surgery Web site. http://www.jcrsjournal.org/content/authorinfo#info. Accessed September 1, 2016.

16. Author Information Pack. American Academy of Ophthalmology Web site. https://www.elsevier.com/wps/find/journaldescription.cws_home/620418?generatepdf=true. Accessed January 19, 2016.

17. Hoffart L, Proust H, Matonti F, Conrath J, Ridings B. Correction of postkeratoplasty astigmatism by femtosecond laser compared with mechanized astigmatic keratotomy. *Am J Ophthalmol.* 2009;147(5):779-787.

18. Wang L, Misra M, Koch DD. Peripheral corneal relaxing incisions combined with cataract surgery. *J Cataract Refract Surg.* 2003;29(4):712-722.

19. Alpins N, Stamatelatos G. Clinical outcomes of laser in situ keratomileusis using combined topography and refractive wavefront treatments for myopic astigmatism. *J Cataract Refract Surg.* 2008;34(8):1250-1259.

20. Gan D, Zhou X, Dai J, et al. Outcomes of epi-LASIK for the correction of high myopia and myopic astigmatism after more than 1 year. *Ophthalmologica.* 2009;223(2):102-110.

21. Alpins NA, Taylor HR, Kent DG, et al. Three multizone photorefractive keratectomy algorithms for myopia. The Melbourne Excimer Laser Group. *J Refract Surg.* 1997;13(6):535-544.

22. Febbraro JL, ron-Rosa D, Gross M, Aron B, Bremond-Gignac D. One year clinical results of photoastigmatic refractive keratectomy for compound myopic astigmatism. *J Cataract Refract Surg.* 1999;25(7):911-920.

23. Taylor HR, Guest CS, Kelly P, Alpins NA. Comparison of excimer laser treatment of astigmatism and myopia. The Excimer Laser and Research Group. *Arch Ophthalmol.* 1993;111(12):1621-1626.

24. Arbelaez MC, Alpins N, Verma S, Stamatelatos G, Arbelaez JG, Arba-Mosquera S. Clinical outcomes of LASIK with an aberration-neutral profile centred on the corneal vertex comparing vector planning to manifest refraction planning for the treatment of myopic astigmatism. *J Cataract Refract Surg.* In press.

25. Morcillo-Laiz R, Zato MA, Munoz-Negrete FJ, rnalich-Montiel F. Surgically induced astigmatism after biaxial phacoemulsification compared to coaxial phacoemulsification. *Eye (Lond).* 2009;23(4):835-839.

26. Alio JL, Agdeppa MC, Pongo VC, El KB. Microincision cataract surgery with toric intraocular lens implantation for correcting moderate and high astigmatism: pilot study. *J Cataract Refract Surg.* 2010;36(1):44-52.

27. Alio JL, Pinero DP, Tomas J, Plaza AB. Vector analysis of astigmatic changes after cataract surgery with implantation of a new toric multifocal intraocular lens. *J Cataract Refract Surg.* 2011;37(7):1217-1229.

28. Galway G, Drury B, Cronin BG, Bourke RD. A comparison of induced astigmatism in 20- vs 25-gauge vitrectomy procedures. *Eye (Lond).* 2010;24(2):315-317.

29. Mountford J, Pesudovs K. An analysis of the astigmatic changes induced by accelerated orthokeratology. *Clin Exp Optom.* 2002;85(5):284-293.

30. Alio JL, Alpins N. Excimer laser correction of astigmatism: consistent terminology for better outcomes. *J Refract Surg.* 2014;30(5):294-295.

31. Alpins N. Vector analysis with the femtosecond laser [letter]. *J Cataract Refract Surg.* 2014;40(7):1246-1247.

32. Pinero DP. Terminology and referencing of astigmatic vector analysis [letter]. *J Cataract Refract Surg.* 2013;39(11):1792.

33. Dupps WJ, Jr. Impact of citation practices: beyond journal impact factors [editorial]. *J Cataract Refract Surg.* 2008;34(9):1419-1421.

34. Alpins N. Astigmatism terminology and source references [letter]. *J Cataract Refract Surg.* 2016;42(4):643.

35. Kunert KS, Russmann C, Blum M, Sluyterman VLG. Vector analysis of myopic astigmatism corrected by femtosecond refractive lenticule extraction. *J Cataract Refract Surg.* 2013;39(5):759-769.

36. St Clair RM, Sharma A, Huang D et al. Development of a nomogram for femtosecond laser astigmatic keratotomy for astigmatism after keratoplasty. *J Cataract Refract Surg.* 2016;42(4):556-562.

37. Trivizki O, Levinger E, Levinger S. Correction ratio and vector analysis of femtosecond laser arcuate keratotomy for the correction of post-mushroom profile keratoplasty astigmatism. *J Cataract Refract Surg.* 2015;41(9):1973-1979.

38. Schallhorn S, Brown M, Venter J, Teenan D, Hettinger K, Yamamoto H. Early clinical outcomes of wavefront-guided myopic LASIK treatments using a new-generation Hartmann-Shack aberrometer. *J Refract Surg.* 2014;30(1):14-21.

39. Koch DD. Astigmatism analysis: the spectrum of approaches [editorial]. *J Cataract Refract Surg.* 2006;32(12):1977-1978.

40. Kanellopoulos AJ. Topography-modified refraction (TMR): adjustment of treated cylinder amount and axis to the topography versus standard clinical refraction in myopic topography-guided LASIK. *Clin Ophthalmol.* 2016;10:2213-2221.

41. Alpins N. Topography-modified refraction: adjustment of treated cylinder amount and axis to the topography versus standard clinical refraction in myopic topography-guided LASIK. *Clinical Ophthalmology.* In press.

42. Alpins N, Stamatelatos G. Customized photoastigmatic refractive keratectomy using combined topographic and refractive data for myopia and astigmatism in eyes with forme fruste and mild keratoconus. *J Cataract Refract Surg.* 2007;33(4):591-602.

43. Alpins N, Stamatelatos G. *Asymmetrical surgical treatment using vector planning.* In: Wang M, ed. Thorofare, NJ: SLACK Incorporated; 2008:263-268.

44. Koch DD. Excimer laser technology: new options coming to fruition [editorial]. *J Cataract Refract Surg.* 1997;23(10):1429-1430.

45. Koch DD. Reporting astigmatism data [editorial]. *J Cataract Refract Surg.* 1998;24(12):1545.

46. Koch DD. How should we analyze astigmatic data? [editorial]. *J Cataract Refract Surg.* 2001;27(1):1-3.

47. Naeser K. Surgically induced astigmatism: distinguishing between dioptric vectors and non-vectors [letter]. *J Refract Surg.* 2015;31(5):349-350.

Chapter 21

Coupling Concepts

LEARNING A COUPLE OF THINGS

The term *coupling* as it applies to the cornea appears to have emerged in the 1970s, although its originator remains obscure. The concept, however, clearly ran through the work of Troutman,[1,2] Thornton,[3,4] Nordan,[5] Buzard,[6] and Binder[7] between 1970 and 1992. Many foundational papers on corneal coupling are included in our 2014 article[8] in the *Journal of Cataract & Refractive Surgery*.

The early definitions of coupling, predictably, arose from the use of incisions— wedge resections[1,2] (Figure 21-1) or relaxing incisions[4] (Figure 21-2), which steepened or flattened the treatment meridian, respectively, in compliance with Gauss's law of elastic domes. The ideal coupling ratio (flattening to steepening) of these incisional approaches is about 1:1, a situation readily demonstrated with the tennis ball cut in half shown in Figure 21-3, where the full amount of flattening at the treatment meridian results in steepening at the opposite meridian after incisional surgery.

LIMITATIONS OF GAUSS'S LAW OF ELASTIC DOMES

A number of authors described useful measures related to changes in the globe from incisional interventions.[9-15] The first measure was coupling (C_{RF}), defined as "the ratio of the magnitude of corneal flattening or steepening in the axis of surgery divided by the magnitude of flattening or steepening 90° away." The same authors described the coupling ratio (CR_{RF}) as "the sphere component in the plus-cylinder refraction divided by the sphere component in the minus-cylinder refraction."[14]

Faktorovich et al[10] later defined two other measures to quantify coupling in arcuate astigmatic keratotomy: the coupling ratio (CR_{FMP}), which is "the flattening of the incised meridian to the steepening of the opposite meridian," 90° to the incised meridian; and the coupling constant (CC_{FMP}), which is "the ratio of the change in spherical equivalent to the magnitude of the vector change in astigmatism" (Figure 21-4). This was effective for incisional surgery but was not useful in identifying the change in laser refractive surgery.

Alpins N. *Practical Astigmatism:
Planning and Analysis* (pp 165-171).
© 2018 SLACK Incorporated.

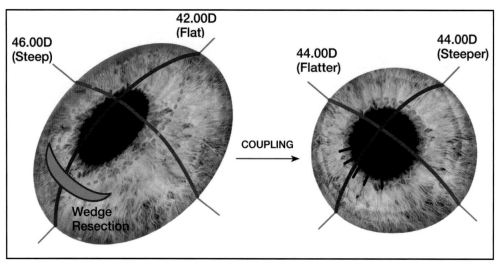

Figure 21-1. A wedge resection on the flat treatment meridian (left), tightened with a number of sutures (right), steepens the flat meridian postkeratoplasty, ideally on a 1:1 ratio that results in an unchanged spherical equivalent.[1,2]

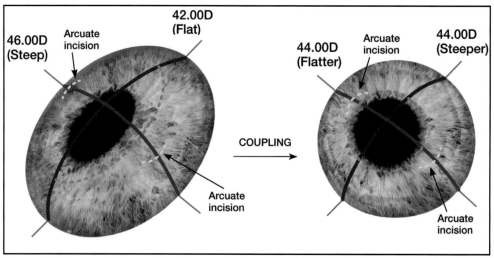

Figure 21-2. Arcuate incisions, a familiar type of refractive surgical incision, flatten the steep treatment meridian and steepen the meridian 90° away, ideally on a 1:1 ratio.[3,4]

In the context of laser ablative surgery, however, the ingenious and tremendously helpful Gaussian law of elastic domes of necessity needed to be left behind. A laser ablation meant that it was then possible to have zero effect in corneal curvature 90° away from the meridian of maximum treatment (the treated steep meridian). Since the CR_{FMP} and C_{RF} as then described would require division by a zero denominator, suddenly, a new solution was needed—one that could take both incisional and ablative corneal changes into account.

Enter the Alpins Method (Figure 21-5).

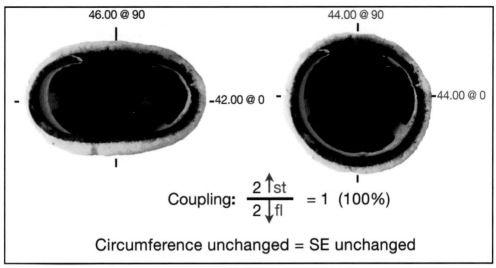

Figure 21-3. A tennis ball, cut in half for demonstration purposes, readily shows the approximate 1:1 ratio of Gauss's law of elastic domes. A 2 D flattening at 90° postoperatively translates to a 2 D steepening at 0° and returns to normal, with no change in circumference, in the absence of compression. This emulates incisional surgery with 100% coupling where there is no change in spherical equivalent.

New Coupling Measures

The Coupling Ratio

Our 2014 paper[8] on corneal coupling details how the Alpins coupling paradigm is valid for both incisional and ablative procedures. A key advance was the observation that the coupling ratio (CR) as we define it *is the change in opposite meridian divided by the change in treatment meridian*, as shown in Figure 21-6—in other words, an important variation from that described by Faktorovich et al.[10] As the reciprocal of the measures used by CR_{FMP} and C_{RF}, the CR was chosen specifically so that it would be meaningful when there is no change at the opposite meridian, which is the usual aim of laser ablation astigmatism treatment.

The Coupling Adjustment

We also introduced the concept of the coupling adjustment (CAdj). The CAdj is the necessary spherical adjustment required as a result of an astigmatic treatment. Our 2014 paper considered how to calculate the measures for compound astigmatic surgical treatments intended to concurrently steepen or flatten the cornea in addition to treating astigmatism. In that publication, the treatment meridian is the axis of the target induced astigmatism vector (TIA)[16] if the treatment is intended to cause local corneal steepening; the meridian 90° away from the treatment meridian is then the opposite meridian. If the intended treatment is to cause local corneal flattening, the treatment meridian is 90° from the axis of the TIA.

The surgically induced astigmatism vector (SIA), as shown in Figure 21-5, is often overestimated in cases where the intended treatment does not line up with the achieved

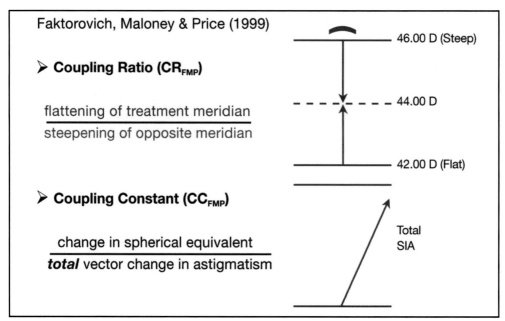

Figure 21-4. CR_{FMP} for incisional astigmatic keratotomy was defined as shown here, and was approximately a 1:1 ratio. The blue arrow simply shows the change between preoperative and postoperative keratometry at the treatment meridian; the red arrow shows an approximately equivalent change in the steepening of the meridian 90° away from the treatment meridian. The coupling constant at this time was defined by the change in spherical equivalent divided by the total vector change in astigmatism, or total SIA.[10]

treatment, as off-axis effect reduces the SIA at the intended treatment meridian. We are interested in the *effective* SIA clinically, as this is the effect at the intended meridian. In cases of regular astigmatism, it is possible to determine the preoperative and postoperative keratometric values at the treatment meridian and opposite meridian by vectorially resolving the measured keratometric astigmatism to these meridians.[17]

A MEANINGFUL APPROACH FOR BOTH ABLATION AND INCISIONAL SURGERY

Our redefined measures of coupling apply both to ablative and incisional approaches. No longer is an arbitrary decision required with coupling related to incisions; namely, whether the change at the surgical treatment meridian should be the numerator or the denominator of the CR. With our proposed approach, a typical laser ablation treatment of astigmatism would have a CR of zero (0% coupling) and a typical limbal relaxing or arcuate incision would have a CR of 1.0 (100% coupling). In contrast, CR_{FMP} and C_{RF} produce infinite values for typical laser ablation treatments of astigmatism, which makes it difficult to evaluate how much a particular treatment deviates from the norm and complicates subsequent analysis of coupling. A coupling ratio of infinity can still occur with our definition, although it would be uncommon; it would occur when there is neither a flattening nor steepening effect at the treatment meridian.

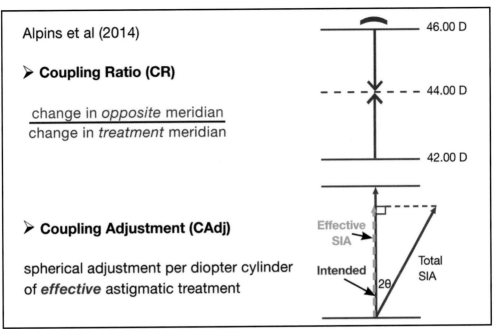

Figure 21-5. CR is defined in our 2014 paper.[8] The CAdj is the spherical adjustment per diopter of cylinder of the effective astigmatic treatment. As implied by the green line, the effective SIA is often overestimated in cases where the intended treatment does not line up with the achieved treatment—any off-axis effect reduces the SIA at the intended treatment meridian by employing only its projected value at the axis of the TIA.

The results derived from keratometric measurements are fundamentally different from those derived from manifest refractive measurements. For example, the effect of a spherical myopic ablation is nonlinearly related to keratometric change but linearly related to refractive change. We know that any post-ablation measurement of corneal power based on anterior corneal curvature only must be incorrect, because there is now a changed relationship between the curvatures of the anterior corneal surface and posterior corneal surface as the curvature of the posterior surface has not changed.[18,19] In the future, it might be preferable to analyze total corneal power data derived from both the anterior and posterior corneal surface.

Because the results from keratometry and refraction are so different, it is important not to mix corneal values and refractive values when calculating coupling measurements. In our analysis of pure spherical ablations, we found that the keratometric change is typically less than the refractive change. Before any analysis of coupling is undertaken, the spherical component of the treatment must be removed from the equation.

ADJUSTING LASER TREATMENT PARAMETERS

Many ophthalmologists adjust treatment parameters that are fed into refractive lasers in an attempt to compensate for consistent over- or undercorrections. We consider these coupling adjustments the same way. The aim is to make the actual treatment as close as

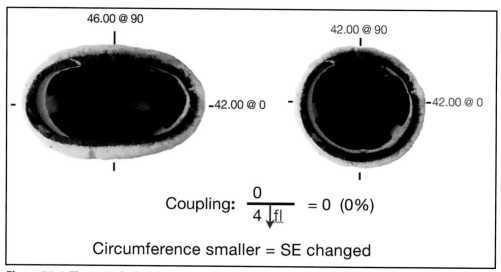

46.00 @ 90

42.00 @ 90

-42.00 @ 0

-42.00 @ 0

Coupling: $\dfrac{0}{4 \downarrow fl} = 0 \ (0\%)$

Circumference smaller = SE changed

Figure 21-6. The tennis ball analogy again shows no change in the keratometry at the opposite meridian. Therefore, there is zero coupling and the spherical equivalent has changed due to a change in the circumference of the tennis ball.

possible to the intended treatment. In fact, only a calibrated laser (with a correct nomogram) will be able to consistently achieve the expected CR of zero. Coupling analysis can determine whether a laser achieves this goal or consistently causes unexpected amounts of coupling.

Similarly, the use of negative cylinder profiles when treating compound hyperopic astigmatism requires the laser to compensate for the fact that the periphery of the cornea is ablated at a different rate than the center of the cornea.[20,21] Although we assume that the profile used has been selected to target the desired refractive treatment effect, coupling analysis can help determine how well a negative cylinder profile treats compound hyperopic astigmatism and how much extra hyperopic spherical treatment it delivers as a result. ASSORT (Alpins Statistical System for Ophthalmic Refractive surgery Techniques) offers a free online coupling calculator (www.assort.com), which can be used to conduct a coupling analysis on any patient.

ISOLATING THE VARIABLES

Ophthalmologists attempting to plan and/or assess the effects of refractive surgery on patients needing both spherical and astigmatic correction face a situation not unlike that seen in studies of nutrition: the difficulty in isolating the various factors that may confound results. It is important to remove the spherical component of the treatment before proceeding with the coupling analysis. Fortunately, the Alpins Method includes coupling concepts,[8] which offer a systematic way to separately analyze the spherical and astigmatic effects of refractive surgery.

Using this approach, it is evident that, when SIA is 45° off, it has no coupling effect. When SIA goes past 45°, the coupling is going in the opposite direction. If you do not use coupling analysis, you are not sure of why you get what you get.

REFERENCES

1. Troutman RC. Control of corneal astigmatism in cataract and corneal surgery. Trans Pac Coast Otoophthalmol Soc Annu Meet. 1970;51:217-231.

2. Troutman RC. Microsurgical control of corneal astigmatism in cataract and keratoplasty. *Trans Am Acad Ophthalmol Otolaryngol.* 1973;77(5):OP563-OP572.

3. Thornton SP. Thornton guide for radial keratotomy incisions and optical zone size (appendix 5-2). In: Sanders DR, Hofmann RF, eds. *Refractive Surgery: A Text of Radial Keratotomy.* Thorofare, NJ: SLACK Incorporated;1985.

4. Thornton SP. Astigmatic keratotomy: a review of basic concepts with case reports. *J Cataract Refract Surg.* 1990;16(4):430-435.

5. Nordan LT. Quantifiable astigmatism correction: concepts and suggestions, 1986. *J Cataract Refract Surg.* 1986;12(5):507-518.

6. Buzard KA, Haight D, Troutman R. Ruiz procedure for postkeratoplasty astigmatism. *J Refract Surg.* 1987;3:40-45.

7. Binder PS, Waring GO. Keratotomy for astigmatism. In: Waring GO, ed. *Refractive Keratotomy for Myopia and Astigmatism.* St. Louis, MO: Mosby-Year Book; 1996:1085-1198.

8. Alpins N, Ong JKY, Stamatelatos G. Corneal coupling of astigmatism applied to incisional and ablative surgery. *J Cataract Refract Surg.* 2014;40:1813-1827.

9. Arbelaez MC, Vidal C, Arba-Mosquera S. Excimer laser correction of moderate to high astigmatism with a non-wavefront-guided aberration-free ablation profile: Six-month results. *J Cataract Refract Surg.* 2009;35(10):1789-1798.

10. Faktorovich EG, Maloney RK, Price FW, Jr. Effect of astigmatic keratotomy on spherical equivalent: results of the Astigmatism Reduction Clinical Trial. *Am J Ophthalmol.* 1999;127(3):260-269.

11. Feizi S, Javadi MA. Corneal graft curvature change after relaxing incisions for post-penetrating keratoplasty astigmatism. *Cornea.* 2012;31(9):1023-1027.

12. Khokhar S, Lohiya P, Murugiesan V, Panda A. Corneal astigmatism correction with opposite clear corneal incisions or single clear corneal incision: comparative analysis. *J Cataract Refract Surg.* 2006;32(9):1432-1437.

13. Moshirfar M, Christiansen SM, Kim G. Comparison of the ratio of keratometric change to refractive change induced by myopic ablation. *J Refract Surg.* 2012;28(10):675-682.

14. Rowsey JJ, Fouraker BD. Corneal coupling principles. *Int Ophthalmol Clin.* 1996;36(4):29-38.

15. Venter J, Blumenfeld R, Schallhorn S, Pelouskova M. Non-penetrating femtosecond laser intrastromal astigmatic keratotomy in patients with mixed astigmatism after previous refractive surgery. *J Refract Surg.* 2013;29(3):180-186.

16. Alpins NA. A new method of analyzing vectors for changes in astigmatism. *J Cataract Refract Surg.* 1993;19(4):524-533.

17. Alpins NA. Vector analysis of astigmatism changes by flattening, steepening, and torque. *J Cataract Refract Surg.* 1997;23(10):1503-1514.

18. Koch DD, Wang L. Calculating IOL power in eyes that have had refractive surgery. *J Cataract Refract Surg.* 2003;29(11):2039-2042.

19. Shammas HJ, Shammas MC, Garabet A, Kim JH, Shammas A, LaBree L. Correcting the corneal power measurements for intraocular lens power calculations after myopic laser in situ keratomileusis. *Am J Ophthalmol.* 2003;136(3):426-432.

20. Arba-Mosquera S, de OD. Geometrical analysis of the loss of ablation efficiency at non-normal incidence. *Opt Express.* 2008;16(6):3877-3895.

21. Mrochen M, Jankov M, Bueeler M, Seiler T. Correlation between corneal and total wavefront aberrations in myopic eyes. *J Refract Surg.* 2003;19(2):104-112.

Chapter 22

Mixed Astigmatism

A Strain on the Brain

The refractive surgical treatment of mixed astigmatism is a challenge, not unlike the brain teaser you may have encountered as a student in math class, where two trains leave two stations traveling at different speeds for different distances, and you must figure their starting times to arrive at the same destination at the same moment—or similar scenarios (see Sidebar 22-1). For many, this type of brain teaser, possibly only encountered in an algebra or trigonometry class, can be a real headache and is typically much more easily solved using a calculator and a clear rationale.

Mixed astigmatism is present when the manifest refraction shows a magnitude of cylinder greater than that of the sphere and having the opposite sign. The optical situation is one in which focal lines from two different meridia straddle the retina, with one (myopic) image focused in front of the retina and one (hyperopic) image focused at a line behind the retina (Figure 22-1). The challenge is to move the images, respectively, backward and forward to coincide squarely at a point on the retina.

Not only is the treatment required to push one image plane back onto the retina and the other image plane forward onto the retina, but this must be done in such a precise manner that differing nomograms adjusting for both positive and negative treatment cylinder effect on the spherical component are necessary (known as the coupling adjustment [CAdj] as described in Chapter 21). This is not trivial, as flattening and steepening ablative treatments—both of which are required in this group of patients—produce different coupling effects and thus, different amounts of spherical shift, usually in opposite spherical directions. (Note—Coupling effects, and concepts such as *coupling ratio* and *coupling adjustment*, are described in Chapter 21 and in greater detail in our 2014 paper.[1])

Clinical Manifestations

We find mixed astigmatism in about 12% of our laser refractive surgery patients. These are often people who have a spherical equivalent not far from zero and may get by often without glasses or with minor vision difficulties more evident at night. Their

Alpins N. *Practical Astigmatism:*
Planning and Analysis (pp 173-178).
© 2018 SLACK Incorporated.

Sidebar 22-1
Planes, Trains, and Autorefractors

Word problems involving trains usually go something like this:

A set of parallel train tracks is 400 miles long. On one end of the track, Train X leaves the station at 5 pm. On the opposite end of the track, Train Y leaves another station at 6:30 pm. If Train A travels 40 mph and Train B travels 60 mph, what time will they meet?

Problems involving multiple distances (D), speeds (S), and times (T) can be difficult to solve because there are many variables. The student wishing to find a solution needs to keep these basic relationships in mind:

- $D = S \times T$
- $S = D \div T$
- $T = D \div S$

When you know any 2 of these quantities, you can solve for the third.

For objects moving in opposite directions toward one another, the sum of their speeds is equal to the speed at which the distance between the objects decreases. In the above example, if Train A and Train B are moving toward each other at 40 mph and 60 mph respectively, then the distance between them is shrinking at a rate of 100 mph.

In any case, the train problem is not dissimilar from the situation the clinician faces when planning an approach to the excimer laser treatment of mixed astigmatism. The disparate images between sphere and cylinder need to be resolved to the plane of the retina, with the least possible stress on the brain for all involved. Fortunately, the ASSORT (Alpins Statistical System for Ophthalmic Refractive surgery Techniques) program includes features to plan and analyze the treatment of mixed astigmatism, and ASSORT offers a free online coupling calculator on its website (www.ASSORT.com).

The train scenarios actually have many analogies in patients with mixed astigmatism. The trains may be leaving different stations (hyperopic vs myopic cylinder) at different times (diopters of cylinder). One might even consider the coupling adjustment as the relative speeds and/or distances involved change, or the point of meeting is shifted. The clinician, of course, wants to end up with a net zero refractive error (trains arriving at the same preferred place at the same time). To do this, the clinician needs to know how the laser is performing and "track" his or her results over time to make the necessary adjustments.

The train scenarios also have many analogies in vector analysis. As described in detail throughout this book, a vector has both a magnitude and a direction. Geometrically, we can picture a vector as a directed line segment, whose length is the magnitude of the vector and, in some cases, an arrow indicating the direction (the direction of the vector from its tail to its head).

And because they can be headaches, most vector calculations remain safely in the background performed by software.

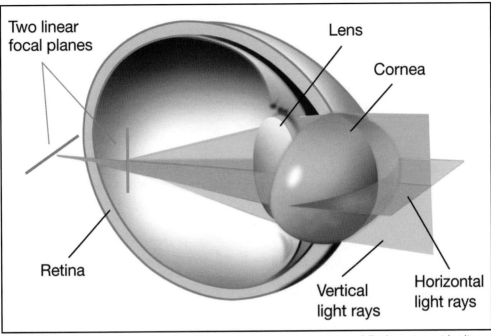

Figure 22-1. In mixed astigmatism, focal lines from 2 different meridia straddle the retina, with 1 linear image in front and the other behind the retina. In this example, the cylinder power at –4.00 D axis 90° exceeds the spherical power at +3.00 D.

unaided visual acuities can measure 20/40 or 20/50. They can drive at night, albeit a bit dangerously. They sometimes get headaches during extended use of their eyes and may complain about not being able to use a computer for extended periods due to vision problems. Glasses often help these patients.

The mixed-astigmatism group of patients can include people with high cylinder where the unaided visual acuity is significantly less than 20/50. Mixed-astigmatism patients considering refractive surgery often have the expected bowtie shape on their corneal topography; the mixed astigmatism is revealed only by a manifest refraction. You may measure refractively a +1.00 D in sphere, with a higher opposite cylinder; for example, a –3.00 D.

CONFOUNDING LASER CONFIGURATIONS

The crux of treating mixed astigmatism relates to the most efficient laser ablation profile. To treat the +1.00 D sphere and –3.00 D cylinder separately removes excess tissue. When the cylinder magnitude is greater than the spherical correction, the surgeon needs to be cognizant of coupling effects and adjustments. It is also important for manufacturers and surgeons to communicate in terms of ablation profiles and any "automatic" treatment parameters where adjustments have been made in the background and are not completely transparent to the surgeon. Depending on the laser and surgeon effects, differences can exist between myopic and hyperopic effects, not necessarily cancelling each other out because of different astigmatism amounts and effects.

Table 22-1 Tissue Ablation —Spherocylinder vs Planocylinder			
Spherocylinder Tx	+1.00 / -2.50 x 90	+1.75 / -3.50 x 90	+3.25 / -5.00 x 90
Spherocylinder Tissue ablated (μm)	28	39	55
Planocylinder Tx Corneal plane +ve 5.0–9.0mm -ve 6.5 x 6.0mm	Plano / +1.22 x 180 Plano / -1.77 x 90	Plano / +2.13 x 180 Plano / -2.07 x 90	Plano / +3.76 x 180 Plano / -2.36 x 90
Planocylinder Tissue ablated (μm)	20	23	34

The most efficient treatment profile for mixed astigmatism in terms of the amount of tissue ablated appears to be bitoric[2-4] (Table 22-1). Plano/positive cylinder and plano/negative cylinder treatments are often programmed into lasers. Some lasers are transparent in allowing the surgeon to customize plus and minus cylinder corrections and some do not; it is preferable to have the ability to modify these settings according to the surgeon's preference and calculated nomograms, in addition to whatever "automatic" modes are preset by the manufacturer.

Figure 22-2 compares spherocylindrical with planocylindrical ablation profiles for mixed astigmatism. In addition to bitoric profiles, other treatment paradigms for mixed astigmatism include cross-cylinder followed by spherical equivalent, and positive cylinder followed by negative sphere. Bitoric appears to be the most common and efficient configuration.

A RETROSPECTIVE CLINICAL STUDY

We've empirically derived the individual coupling adjustments of the myopic and hyperopic cylindrical components of a bitoric treatment to compare the theoretical combined treatment effect on spherical equivalent to the actual change in refractive spherical equivalent using the ViSX STAR S4 IR excimer laser (Johnson & Johnson).[5] The coupling adjustments that provided the best fit in both mean and standard deviation were considered the historical coupling adjustments. Theoretical treatments that incorporated the historical coupling adjustments were then calculated. This allowed us to compare the distribution of postoperative spherical equivalent errors and the theoretically adjusted distribution.

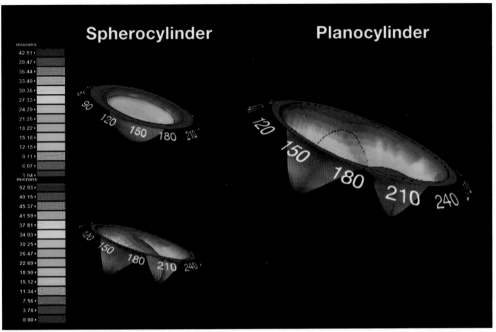

Figure 22-2. A planocylindrical tissue ablation appears to remove less tissue than the spherocylindrical profile.

We found a myopic coupling adjustment that was virtually nil (-0.02); however, the hyperopic coupling adjustment was 0.30. This implies that almost no adjustment of the myopic component of the bitoric treatment was necessary, but that the hyperopic component of the bitoric treatment generated a large amount of unintended spherical (myopic) shift. The theoretically adjusted treatments targeted zero mean spherical equivalent error, as intended, and the distribution of the theoretical spherical equivalent errors had the same spread as the distribution of actual postoperative spherical equivalent errors. To us, this means that historical coupling adjustments for both myopic and hyperopic cylinder together should be taken into consideration when planning mixed-astigmatism treatments in order to improve surgical results.

TWEEZING THE SPHERICAL FROM THE CYLINDRICAL

Our approach is to assess the spherical and cylindrical treatment components in these patients separately. We want to narrow the bell-shaped curve, and to shift it from a bias for hyperopia to a bias for myopia—ideally, to shift it to zero. If you do not separate the spherical from the cylindrical components, you really do not know exactly what your surgery is doing. Over time—perhaps with a few hundred patients—a nomogram can be developed to prevent over- or undercorrection of the spherical equivalent and a coupling adjustment of cylinder to sphere can be incorporated into the treatment plan. I think that unique surgeon-related, environmental, and other factors exist that will make it difficult for manufacturers to initiate a "standard" general nomogram adjustment for coupling, and that it will always be important for surgeons to calculate these adjustments for themselves.

REFERENCES

1. Alpins N, Ong JKY, Stamatelatos G. Corneal coupling of astigmatism applied to incisional and ablative surgery. *J Cataract Refract Surg.* 2014;40:1813-1827.

2. Azar DT, Primack JD. Theoretical analysis of ablation depths and profiles in laser in situ keratomileusis for compound hyperopic and mixed astigmatism. *J Cataract Refract Surg.* 2000;26(8):1123-1136.

3. de Ortueta D, Arba-Mosquera S, Haecker C. Treating mixed astigmatism: a theoretical comparison and guideline for combined ablation strategies and wavefront ablation. In: Goggin M, ed. *Astigmatism: Optics, Physology and Management*. Rijeka, Croatia: InTech; 2012:125-134.

4. Gatinel D, Hoang-Xuan T, Azar DT. Three-dimensional representation and qualitative comparisons of the amount of tissue ablation to treat mixed and compound astigmatism. *J Cataract Refract Surg.* 2002;28(11):2026-2034.

5. Alpins N, Ong JKY, Stamatelatos G. Planning for coupling effects in bitoric mixed astigmatism ablative treatments. *J Refract Surg.* In press.

Chapter 23

How to Perform Your Own Corneal and Refractive Vector Analyses

INDIVIDUAL ANALYSIS BASED ON PREOPERATIVE AND POSTOPERATIVE REFRACTION

One of the most common questions that a refractive surgeon will want to answer is whether the procedure successfully addresses, not only the refractive astigmatism, but the corneal astigmatism as well. The analyses that should be performed are a comparison between the intended change in refractive cylinder and the actual effect of the surgery on the refractive cylinder and the intended change in corneal astigmatism and the actual change.[1] In most cases of excimer laser surgery, the intended change in astigmatism is quantified by the target induced astigmatism vector (TIA) by refraction, and the actual astigmatic effect is quantified by the surgically induced astigmatism vector (SIA) by refraction and by corneal astigmatism. The difference vector (DV) by refraction and by corneal values is the amount that the actual effect of the surgery missed the intended refractive cylindrical or corneal target.

This type of analysis is suitable for most surgical refractive procedures. However, this sort of analysis should not be used to quantify the effects of refractive cataract surgery with toric lens implantation—a hybrid analysis (described later) is more appropriate.

The first step is to shift the refractive powers to the desired reference plane, which is typically the corneal plane for a corneal or intraocular procedure. Lens power F_{SP} at the spectacle plane with back vertex distance (BVD) in millimeters can be shifted to lens power F_{CP} at the corneal plane by using the formula

$$F_{CP} = 1/\left(\frac{1}{F_{SP}} - \frac{BVD}{1000}\right)$$

For spherocylindrical refractions, the lens powers for the two principal meridia are shifted separately.

The next step is to calculate the surgical vectors—TIA, SIA, and DV—by refraction. This is most easily illustrated on a double-angle vector diagram (DAVD) (Figure 23-1). The preoperative, postoperative, and target refractive cylinders at the corneal plane

Alpins N. *Practical Astigmatism:
Planning and Analysis* (pp 179-196).
© 2018 SLACK Incorporated.

Figure 23-1. Graphical representation of individual vector analysis by refraction.

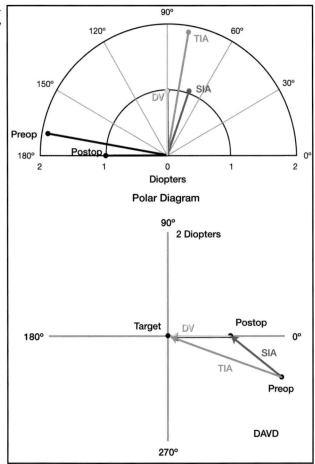

have magnitude equal to the cylinder magnitude, and orientation of twice the positive cylinder axis. The double-angle vector for the TIA by refraction starts at the preoperative refractive cylinder and ends at the target refractive cylinder. Similarly, the double-angle vector for the SIA by refraction starts at the preoperative refractive cylinder and ends at the postoperative refractive cylinder. The double-angle vector for the DV points from the postoperative refractive cylinder to the target refractive cylinder. To convert the TIA, SIA, and DV back to polar form (with axis between 0° and 180°), simply halve the axis of the double-angle vector while keeping the same magnitude.

There are 4 summary statistics that can highlight different aspects of the SIA, TIA, and DV. The correction index (CI) is the SIA magnitude divided by the TIA magnitude, and shows whether the actual treatment was an over- or undercorrection, as a proportion of the intended treatment. The index of success (IOS) is the DV magnitude divided by the TIA magnitude, which shows how large the error in treatment was as a proportion of the size of the intended treatment. The magnitude of error (ME) is the SIA magnitude minus the TIA magnitude, and shows the amount of over- or undercorrection in diopters. Finally, the angle of error (AE) is the SIA axis minus the TIA axis, in the range between -90° and 90°. Note that the end point extremes of -90° and 90° actually describe the same AE, and we typically prefer to use 90° instead of -90°.

Example

The data needed to perform this individual analysis are:

Preoperative refraction (BVD: 12 mm)	-1.00 / -2.00 X 80
Target refraction	Plano
Postoperative refraction (BVD: 12 mm)	-0.25 / -1.00 X 90

To shift the preoperative refraction to the corneal plane, we split it up into the 2 principal meridia: -1.00 @ 80 and -3.00 @ 170. Each of these is then shifted:

$$1/\left(\frac{1}{-1.00} - \frac{12}{1000}\right) = -0.99 @ 80$$

$$1/\left(\frac{1}{-3.00} - \frac{12}{1000}\right) = -2.90 @ 170$$

The preoperative refraction at the corneal plane is then recombined into -2.90 / +1.91 X 170. Note that we use positive cylinder form, which is the form required for further analysis.

Similarly, the target refraction at the corneal plane is plano, and the postoperative refraction at the corneal plane is -1.23 / +0.98 X 180.

The polar and double-angle plots in Figure 23-1 show the preoperative, postoperative, and target refractive cylinders, and the SIA, TIA, and DV.

The preoperative cylinder representation on the DAVD, which has magnitude 1.91 and axis 2*170° = 340°, has Cartesian coordinates of x = 1.91 cos 340° = 1.79, y = 1.91 sin 340° = -0.65, or as commonly written (1.79, -0.65). The postoperative cylinder representation on the DAVD has Cartesian coordinates (1.00, 0.00), and the target for this example is at the origin (0.00, 0.00).

The TIA double-angle vector is calculated as the vector difference between the target cylinder and the preoperative cylinder on the DAVD: (0.00, 0.00) – (1.79, -0.65) = (-1.79, 0.65). The SIA double-angle vector is the difference between the postoperative cylinder and the preoperative cylinder on the DAVD: (0.98, 0.00) – (1.79, -0.65) = (-0.81, 0.65). The DV double-angle vector is (0.00, 0.00) – (0.98, 0.00) = (-0.98, 0.00).

To convert the TIA double-angle vector back to polar coordinates, we calculate the magnitude (in diopters) using Pythagoras' theorem: $\sqrt{(-1.79)^2 + 0.65^2} = 1.91$, and the axis is calculated to be half the arctangent: 0.5 * atan2(x = -1.79, y=0.65) = 80°; this is commonly written as 1.91 Ax 80°. Note that it is important to use the atan2 function if calculating this with a computer program so that the result of the arctangent ends up in the correct quadrant. The SIA and DV can be converted back to polar coordinates in the same way: SIA: 1.04 Ax 71°, DV: 0.98 Ax 90°. Note that the TIA, SIA, and DV must always have a positive magnitude. If negative, then the direction must be reversed by 180° on a DAVD.

The correction index is the SIA magnitude divided by the TIA magnitude: CI = 1.04 / 1.91 = 0.55. The index of success is the DV magnitude divided by the TIA magnitude: IOS = 0.98 / 1.91 = 0.51. The magnitude of error is the SIA magnitude minus the TIA magnitude: MoE = 1.04 – 1.91 = -0.87 D. The angle of error is the SIA axis minus the TIA magnitude in the range -90° to 90°: AE = 71 – 80 = -9°.

TIA	1.91 Ax 80
SIA	1.04 Ax 71
DV	0.98 Ax 90
CI	0.55
IOS	0.51
ME	0.87 D
AE	-9°

INDIVIDUAL ANALYSIS BASED ON PREOPERATIVE AND POSTOPERATIVE CORNEAL ASTIGMATISM: A PARALLEL ANALYSIS

A refractive surgeon will often also be interested in the effect of a refractive procedure on the corneal astigmatism, particularly when the patient presents with good visual acuity but is complaining about the quality of vision. For this analysis, the actual change in corneal astigmatism is compared with the expected or intended change in corneal astigmatism.

The actual measurement of corneal astigmatism may be made using a keratometer, topographer, or tomographer. The method of measurement should be reported along with the actual measurements since different methods will give different results. Thus, if the analysis was based on topography, the intended change would be quantified by the TIA which is the actual treatment applied, and the actual astigmatic effect is quantified by the SIA by topography. Note, that each individual analysis should use the same device to measure both the pre- and postoperative corneal astigmatism.

There is only one common TIA for each procedure regardless of whether the analysis is done by refractive or corneal parameters. After the TIA and SIA have been calculated, then the DV is the vectorial difference between the TIA and the SIA. The remaining analysis is then identical to that performed in a refractive analysis, resulting in a CI, IOS, ME, and AE.

Example of Parallel Corneal Analysis

In this example, we will analyze the same eye that was used in the refractive analysis, thus, the TIA is identical to that analysis.

The data needed to perform this individual analysis are:

Preoperative corneal astigmatism (simulated keratometry)	1.70 @ 167
TIA	1.91 Ax 80
Postoperative corneal astigmatism (simulated keratometry)	0.50 @ 30

In the analysis, we will move freely between polar form, which has a magnitude at a certain orientation, and Cartesian form, which is displayed in (x, y) form.

The preoperative corneal astigmatism is 1.70 @ 167 = (1.70 * cos (2*167°), 1.70 * sin (2*167°)) = (1.53, -0.75). The postoperative corneal astigmatism is 0.50 @ 30 = (0.25, 0.43). The TIA is 1.91 Ax 80 = (-1.79, 0.65).

The SIA is the vectorial difference between the postoperative and preoperative corneal astigmatisms: (0.25, 0.43) – (1.53, -0.75) = (-1.28, 1.18) = 1.74 Ax 69.

The target corneal astigmatism is the TIA added vectorially to the preoperative corneal astigmatism: (1.53, -0.75) + (-1.79, 0.65) = (-0.27, -0.09) = 0.28 @ 100.

The DV is the vectorial difference between the postoperative and target corneal astigmatisms: (-0.27, -0.09) – (0.25, 0.43) = (-0.52, -0.52) = 0.74 Ax 113.

The polar and double-angle plots in Figure 23-2 show the preoperative, postoperative, and target refractive cylinders, and the SIA, TIA, and DV.

The CI is the SIA magnitude divided by the TIA magnitude: CI = 1.74 / 1.91 = 0.91. The IOS is the DV magnitude divided by the TIA magnitude: IOS = 0.74 / 1.91 = 0.39. The ME is the SIA magnitude minus the TIA magnitude: MoE = 1.74 – 1.91 = -0.17 D. The AE is the SIA axis minus the TIA magnitude in the range -90° to 90°: AE = 69 – 80 = -11°.

TIA	1.91 Ax 80
SIA	1.74 Ax 69
DV	0.74 Ax 113
CI	0.91
IOS	0.39
ME	-0.17 D
AE	-11°

GROUP ANALYSIS BASED ON PREOPERATIVE AND POSTOPERATIVE REFRACTION OR CORNEAL ASTIGMATISM

A group analysis is necessary when adjusting treatment nomograms. The simplest type of group analysis is to calculate measures of central tendency for everything calculated in the individual analyses.

Figure 23-2. Graphical representation of individual vector analysis by simulated keratometry.

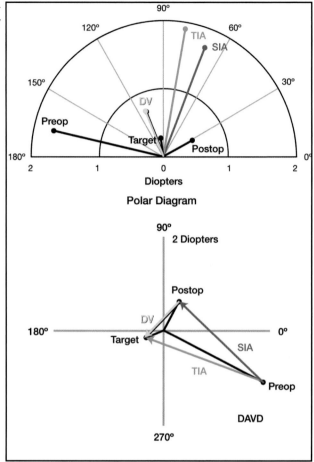

For TIA, SIA, and DV, the appropriate measure of central tendency is a summated vector mean (also known as the centroid). For the CI, a geometric mean is appropriate because it is a ratio that is ideally centered near 1.0. The IOS is also a ratio, but it is always positive and ideally centered near zero; for this, we use a square root mean to normalize the underlying distribution. The arithmetic mean is used for the ME and AE.

To calculate a summated vector mean, the individual vectors in polar coordinates are converted into double-angle vectors, then the x values and y values are both averaged to give the double-angle summated vector mean in Cartesian coordinates. This double-angle summated vector mean is converted back into polar coordinates by halving the axis.

A geometric mean is calculated by taking logarithms of the individual values, calculating the mean of these logarithms, and then taking the antilog of the mean. We show the formula using base-10 logarithms here:

$$10^{\overline{\log_{10} x_i}}$$

where the individual values are x_i.

The square root mean transformation that we use is calculated by taking the square root of the individual values, then calculating the mean of these transformed values, and finally taking the square of the mean:

$$\left(\overline{\sqrt{x_i}} \right)^2$$

where the individual values are x_i.

For a group analysis to be meaningful, the group must be large enough to account for the variation between individuals. Typically, we use a group size of at least 50 for simple analyses, and a larger group size for more complex analyses.

Example of Group Analyses

In this example, we perform a group analysis on 5 cases by refraction to illustrate the calculations required. Naturally, we could also perform a group analysis by corneal astigmatism, which would look almost identical.

The refractive measurements are shown in Table 23-1:

	Preop Rx (BVD 12 mm)	Postop Rx (BVD 12 mm)	Preop Rx (Corneal plane)	Postop Rx (Corneal plane)
Case 1	-1.00 / -2.00 X 80	-0.25 / -1.00 X 90	-0.99 / -1.91 X 80	-0.25 / -0.98 X 90
Case 2	-2.25 / -1.25 X 110	pl / -0.50 X 105	-2.19 / -1.17 X 110	pl / -0.50 X 105
Case 3	-1.75 / -2.25 X 95	+0.25	-1.71 / -2.10 X 95	+0.25
Case 4	-3.25 / -1.00 X 90	+0.25 / -0.25 X 180	-3.13 / -0.92 X 90	+0.25 / -0.25 X 180
Case 5	pl / -4.00 X 93	-0.25 / -0.75 X 85	pl / -3.82 X 93	-0.25 / -0.74 X 85

Table 23-1
Pre- and Postoperative Refractive Measurements for 5 Cases of Excimer Laser Surgery

In all these cases, the refractive target was plano.

The individual analyses are calculated as described previously, with values shown in Table 23-2:

Table 23-2
Astigmatic Analyses of 5 Cases of Excimer Laser Surgery From Table 23-1

	TIA	SIA	DV	CI	IOS	ME(D)	AE (°)
Case 1	1.91 Ax 80	1.04 Ax 71	0.98 Ax 90	0.55	0.51	-0.87	-9
Case 2	1.17 Ax 110	0.68 Ax 114	0.50 Ax 105	0.58	0.43	-0.49	4
Case 3	2.10 Ax 95	2.10 Ax 95	0.00 Ax —	1.00	0.00	0.00	0
Case 4	0.92 Ax 90	1.17 Ax 90	0.25 Ax 180	1.27	0.27	0.25	0
Case 5	3.82 Ax 93	3.12 Ax 95	0.74 Ax 85	0.82	0.19	-0.70	2

The TIA summated vector mean is calculated by converting the TIAs from polar to double-angle Cartesian vectors, finding the mean x and y values of the Cartesian vectors, then converting the resulting average Cartesian vector back to polar form (Table 23-3):

Table 23-3
Double-Angle Cartesian Coordinates of TIA for 5 Cases in Table 23-1

	TIA (Polar)	TIA (Double-Angle Cartesian)
Case 1	1.91 Ax 80	(-1.79, 0.65)
Case 2	1.17 Ax 110	(-0.90, -0.75)
Case 3	2.10 Ax 95	(-2.07, -0.36)
Case 4	0.92 Ax 90	(-0.92, 0.00)
Case 5	3.82 Ax 93	(-3.80, -0.40)

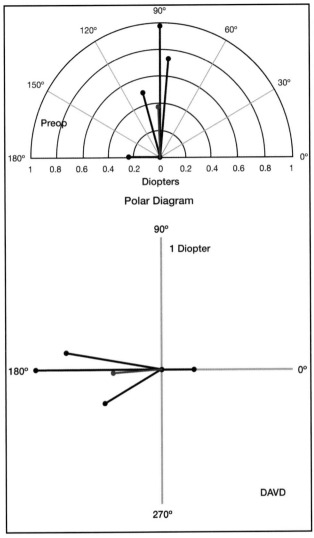

Figure 23-3. Graphical representation of group analysis by refraction. The black lines show the 5 individual difference vectors (1 of which is at the origin), and the red line shows the summated vector mean.

Mean double-angle TIA x value: $((-1.79) + (-0.90) + (-2.07) + (-0.92) + (-3.80)) / 5 = -1.90$.

Mean double-angle TIA y value: $((0.65 + (-0.75) + (-0.36) + 0.00 + (-0.40)) / 5 = -0.17$.

This converts back to the polar form of 1.90 Ax 93. The SIA and DV summated vector means are calculated similarly.

These vectorial group analyses can be displayed on a polar plot or a DAVD. We show the DV group analysis in Figure 23-3.

The CI geometric mean is calculated as

$$10^{(\log_{10} 0.55 + \log_{10} 0.58 + \log_{10} 1.00 + \log_{10} 1.27 + \log_{10} 0.82)} = 0.80$$

The IOS square mean root is calculated as

$$(\sqrt{0.51} + \sqrt{0.43} + \sqrt{0.00} + \sqrt{0.27} + \sqrt{0.19})^2 = 0.22$$

The ME mean is calculated as $((-0.87) + (-0.49) + 0.00 + 0.25 + (-0.70)) / 5 = -0.36$.
The AE mean is calculated similarly: $((-9) + 4 + 0 + 0 + 2) / 5 = -0.6$.

In some cases, it can be useful to calculate the mean of the magnitudes of the AEs, ignoring their sign. This AE absolute mean would be $(9 + 4 + 0 + 0 + 2) / 5 = 3$.

TIA Summated Vector Mean	1.90 Ax 93
SIA summated vector mean	1.52 Ax 93
DV summated vector mean	0.38 Ax 92
CI geometric mean	0.80
IOS square mean root	0.22
ME mean	-0.36 D
AE arithmetic mean	-0.6°
AE absolute mean	3°

INDIVIDUAL ANALYSIS OF CORNEAL INCISIONS

The astigmatic effect of a corneal incision can be quantified by the flattening/steepening and torque components of the corneal SIA.[2] The flattening/steepening component, which is the radial component of the SIA at the position of the incision, characterizes the part of the SIA that changes the magnitude of the corneal astigmatism. The torque component is the tangential component of the SIA, which causes a change in the orientation of the corneal astigmatism, as well as a slight increase in its magnitude. This differs from a pure rotatory component, which would change the orientation, but not the magnitude of the corneal astigmatism.

This type of analysis is typically used to determine the astigmatic effect of limbal relaxing incisions or phacoemulsification incisions. It can be problematic to apply for very large incisions ($>90°$), where the incision is not easily localizable to one particular corneal position and orientation. It is not appropriate to use such an analysis in the case of irregular corneal astigmatism or when the keratometric and topographic measurement of corneal astigmatism is unreliable.

The corneal SIA is the astigmatic difference between the postoperative and preoperative corneal astigmatisms, and is most easily calculated using double-angle analysis (see Figure 23-4). These astigmatisms are represented on a DAVD with the same magnitudes as the original astigmatisms, and oriented at twice the values of the steep meridia. The corneal SIA double-angle vector starts at the preoperative astigmatism and ends at the postoperative astigmatism on a DAVD.

Once the corneal SIA double-angle vector has been calculated, it is resolved into 2 perpendicular double-angle vector components: the flattening/steepening double-angle vector is in the orientation of twice the incision meridian, and the torque double-angle vector is at right angles to that. One of the easiest ways to resolve a vector in a given direction is to multiply the magnitude by the cosine of the angle between the vector orientation and the required direction. For double-angle vector with magnitude C and orientation A, and incision meridian M, the resolved magnitude is

$$\| C \cos (A - M) \|.$$

The resolved component that is perpendicular to that has magnitude is

$$\| C \sin (A - M) \|.$$

The signs of the cosine and sine indicate whether the components are steepening or flattening, and counterclockwise or clockwise, respectively.

The double-angle vectors that have been calculated are converted back to polar notation by keeping the magnitudes unchanged, but halving the axes. Each polar representation is oriented at the actual orientation as it appears on the eye.

Note, that it is also possible to do a refractive analysis of corneal incisions, although this is less common. This is based on the pre- and postoperative refractive cylinders at the corneal plane, represented in positive cylinder form. It may be useful, for example, in a healthy eye with a clear lens undergoing arcuate keratotomy for astigmatism where the spherical equivalent is close to plano.

Example of Corneal Incisional Analysis

The data needed to perform this individual analysis are:

Preoperative corneal astigmatism	1.75 D @ 180 (steep meridian)
Incision Meridian	20°
Postoperative corneal astigmatism	0.65 @ 170 (steep meridian)

Preoperative corneal astigmatism (double-angle): (1.75, 0.00).
Postoperative corneal astigmatism (double-angle): (0.61, -0.22).
The corneal SIA is the double-angle vector difference between the postoperative astigmatism and the preoperative astigmatism: (0.61, -0.22) – (1.75, 0.00) = (-1.14, -0.22). In polar coordinates, this is 1.16 Ax 96.
To calculate the flattening/steepening, the SIA double-angle vector is resolved in the direction of 2*20°. The magnitude is

$$\| 1.16 \cos 2(96° - 20°) \| = 1.02$$

and since the cosine is negative, this indicates that the effect is flattening.

Figure 23-4. Graphical representation of individual analysis of a corneal incision. On the double-angle vector diagram, the flattening is the portion of the SIA parallel to twice the incision meridian, and the torque is the portion of the SIA perpendicular to the flattening.

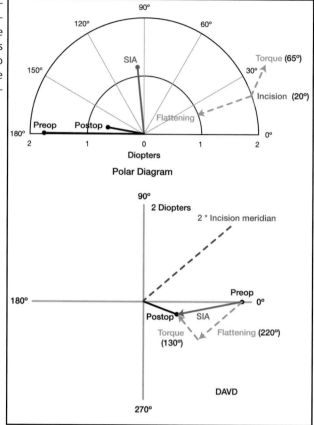

To calculate the torque, the component of the SIA is resolved perpendicular to the flattening/steepening component. The magnitude is

$$\| 1.16 \sin 2(96° - 20°) \| = 0.54$$

and since the sine is positive, this indicates that the effect is counterclockwise torque.

The graphical representation of this analysis is shown in Figure 23-4. We find it useful to display the flattening and torque components at the location of the incision, with a flattening arrow pointing from the incision towards the origin, and the torque pointing in the direction of its polar axis (half the axis on the DAVD). If we had a steepening instead of a flattening, we would represent this as an arrow pointing from the incision directly away from the origin.

SIA	1.16 Ax 96
Flattening	1.02 D
Torque	0.54 D, counterclockwise

GROUP ANALYSIS OF CORNEAL INCISIONS

A group analysis of corneal incisions is usually performed to determine the average flattening/steepening and torque effects of a certain type of incision. Both the flattening/steepening and the torque can be summarized with arithmetic averages. A convention to which we adhere during the group analysis is to indicate flattening with a negative value and steepening with a positive value. We also give clockwise torque a negative value and counterclockwise torque a positive value.

It is important to only aggregate results from incisions that have the same type, depth, and extent, and that are performed at roughly the same position on the eye. Indeed, flattening effects are not necessarily symmetrical between the 2 eyes.[3] Thus, it will be necessary to perform a separate group analysis for each incision type and position. Also, incision effects can differ depending on the amount of preoperative corneal astigmatism, and whether the incision is made on a steep or flat part of the cornea.[3]

From our experience, there should be at least 30 cases (but we prefer 50) in each group to ensure that the group analysis is meaningful, since there is a lot of variance in the flattening/steepening effect of incisions. If the number of cases being analyzed is small, it may be necessary to group incisions together that are at nearby locations on the eye; for example, all left-eye incisions at 350°, 0,° 10°, and 20° into a "left-eye temporal incision" group.

Example

In this example, we show a group analysis on 10 incisions (Table 23-4) to illustrate the calculations required. We will assume that the incisions are all 2.2 mm phacoemul-

Table 23-4
Group Analyses on 10 Incisions to Illustrate the Calculations Required
The Incisions Are All 2.2 mm Phacoemulsification Incisions on Left Eyes

Incision Position (°)	Preoperative Corneal Steep Meridian (°)	Flattening/Steepening Magnitude (D) postive = steepening, negative = flattening	Torque Magnitude (D) positive = counter clockwise, negative = clockwise
0	178	-0.25	0.05
0	0	-0.35	0.03
0	4	-0.20	0.01
10	10	-0.40	-0.02
10	12	-0.28	-0.07
20	15	-0.22	-0.06
20	20	-0.17	0.00
20	30	-0.15	0.10
20	80	0.06	0.21
20	90	-0.02	0.17

sification incisions on left eyes. We will also ignore the magnitude of the preoperative corneal astigmatism, although this could be factored into the grouping if there were more data.

The first step is to decide whether it is necessary to further subdivide this particular group into subgroups (ignoring the fact that a group this small doesn't give meaningful results). One way to divide up the incisions is by incision position; the other way is to classify all the incision positions as temporal, superior, or oblique. It is then necessary to divide the eyes based on whether the corneal astigmatism starts out being with-the-rule, against-the-rule, or oblique.

Here, we will group the incisions by incision position and type of corneal astigmatism (Table 23-5).

| | | Table 23-5 | |
| | | **Incisions in Table 23-4 Are Grouped by Incision Position and Type of Corneal Astigmatism and Then Analyzed** | |
Group	Number of Cases	Mean Flattening/Steepening Magnitude (D)	Mean Torque Magnitude (D)
0° incision, ATR cornea	3	-0.27	0.03
10° incision, ATR cornea	2	-0.34	-0.05
20° incision, ATR cornea	3	-0.18	0.01
20° incision, WTR cornea	2	0.02	0.19

The mean flattening/steepening for incisions at 0° on ATR corneas (with a steep meridian near 0 or 180°) is ((-0.25) + (-0.35) + (-0.20)) / 3 = -0.27. The mean torque for these incisions is (0.05 + 0.03 + 0.01) / 3 = 0.03. The rest of the averages are then calculated similarly.

A graphical overview of the group analysis can be useful to give a quick summary of the results. Figure 23-5 shows the results for the ATR corneas.

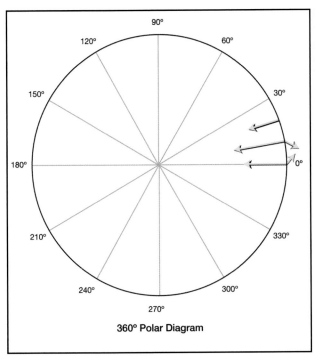

Figure 23-5. Graphical representation of group analysis of corneal incisions. We show the results of incisions at 0°, 10°, and 20° for the against-the-rule corneas in the example. The arrows pointing radially toward the origin represent flattening, while the small arrows outside the circle represent torque.

INDIVIDUAL ANALYSIS OF THE ASTIGMATIC EFFECT OF A TORIC INTRAOCULAR LENS

The analysis necessary to quantify the success of refractive cataract surgery with a toric implant lens can be quite complicated. Here, we deal with the relatively simple case of a small-incision cataract extraction utilizing phacoemulsification and then implantation of a toric intraocular lens (IOL), without the use of additional limbal relaxing incisions.

Since the natural crystalline lens is extracted during the procedure, the preoperative refraction (which includes the effect of the cataractous crystalline lens) doesn't directly provide any useful information for this astigmatic analysis. Instead, the preoperative astigmatic status of the eye is taken to be preoperative corneal astigmatism, with the simplistic assumption (discussed below) that all astigmatism in the aphakic eye is caused by the cornea. The postoperative astigmatic status of the eye is taken to be the postoperative refractive cylinder at the corneal plane.

The effect of the phacoemulsification incision on the corneal astigmatism can be estimated based on previous group analysis, or calculated directly as the difference between the post- and the preoperative corneal astigmatism.

The TIA of the implanted toric lens is the equivalent lens power at the corneal plane. These can be calculated directly by using any multitude of vergence formulas and surgeon constants.[4] However, there are many calculators that perform this calculation, some embedded in measurement devices, others available on the internet. Caution is advised when selecting a calculator to calculate the corneal plane power of an IOL, since some calculators are far too simplistic and assume a fixed ratio between the toric implant power and the TIA at the corneal plane. At a minimum, a toric calculator should consider the corneal power, the axial length, and the spherical equivalent power of the implant, as well as include some customization specific to the lens type; for example, an optimized lens constant for a specific surgeon.

The total refractive change in astigmatism caused by the implanted toric IOL (as quantified by the SIA) can be calculated as the astigmatic difference between the postoperative refractive cylinder and the preoperative corneal astigmatism, excluding the effect of the phacoemulsification incision. Equivalently, this is the astigmatic difference between the postoperative refractive cylinder and the post-incisional corneal astigmatism (assuming that a valid reliable measurement or estimate is possible).

The common assumption that the cornea is the only source of astigmatism in an aphakic eye is easy to understand based on optical principles. However, there also seems to be a non-optical influence on the amount of astigmatism present in the manifest refraction, which may be due to a subjective perception of astigmatism that does not match the optical reality.[5,6] As technology progresses, it may be possible in the future to directly measure the astigmatic effect of the cataractous lens. However, it will still be problematic to achieve a reliable subjective refraction for an eye with a cataract, and this may always be the essential limiting factor in a purely refractive analysis.

Example

The data needed to perform this individual analysis are:

Preoperative corneal astigmatism	1.90 D @ 167
Expected flattening at phaco incision	0.25 D
Position of phaco incision	10°
Toric power of implanted lens at corneal plane	1.54 D X 164
Target refractive cylinder	0.20 D X 164
Postoperative refraction (BVD: 12 mm)	+0.25 / -0.75 X 120
Postoperative refraction (corneal plane)	+0.25 / -0.75 X 120

The data pertaining to the toric lens and the target refractive cylinder are assumed to be taken from a toric calculator.

As in the previous sections, Cartesian double-angle notation is denoted in (x,y) form, while polar notation is a magnitude at a certain orientation.

The post-incisional corneal astigmatism is estimated here as the 1.90 D @ 167 plus 0.25 D flattening @ 10: (1.90 cos 2*167, 1.90 sin 2*167) − (0.25 cos 2*10, 0.25 sin 2*10) = (1.47, -0.92) = 1.74 @ 164.

The postoperative refractive cylinder at the corneal plane is +0.75 X 30 = (0.38, 0.65).

The SIA of the refractive change induced by the toricity of the implant is the difference between the postoperative refractive cylinder and the post-incisional corneal astigmatism: (0.38, 0.65) − (1.47, -0.92) = (-1.10, 1.57) = 1.91 Ax 62.

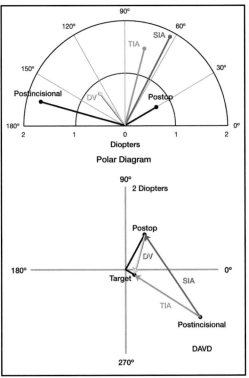

Figure 23-6. Graphical representation of hybrid vector analysis of the astigmatic effect of a toric lens implant.

The TIA is the toric power of the implanted lens at the corneal plane, namely 1.54 Ax 74 = (-1.31, 0.82).

The DV is the vectorial difference between the TIA and the SIA: (-1.31, 0.82) - (-1.10, 1.57) = (-0.21, -0.75) = 0.78 Ax 127.

Figure 23-6 shows a graphical representation of these calculations.

The CI is the refractive SIA magnitude induced by the implant divided by the TIA magnitude: CI = 1.91 / 1.54 = 1.24. The index of success is the DV magnitude divided by the TIA magnitude: IOS = 0.78 / 1.54 = 0.51. The magnitude of error is the SIA magnitude minus the TIA magnitude: MoE = 1.91 − 1.54 = 0.37 D. The angle of error is the SIA axis minus the TIA magnitude in the range -90° to 90°: AE = 62 − 74 = -12°.

TIA	1.54 Ax 74
SIA	1.91 Ax 62
DV	0.78 Ax 127
CI	1.24
IOS	0.51
ME	0.37 D
AE	-12°

GROUP ANALYSIS OF THE ASTIGMATIC EFFECT OF A TORIC IOL

After individual analyses have been performed to determine the astigmatic effect of implanted toric lenses, they can be aggregated in a group analysis. When considering which analyses to group together, the surgeon should consider surgical factors as well as the type and power of IOL being implanted.

The actual procedure of generating a group analysis is identical to that used for the group analysis based on preoperative and postoperative refraction data. The individual TIAs, SIAs, and DVs are summarized by summated vector means, and the various indices are averaged after appropriate transformation to normalize the underlying distributions.

REFERENCES

1. Alpins NA. A new method of analyzing vectors for changes in astigmatism. *J Cataract Refract Surg.* 1993;19(4):524-533.
2. Alpins NA. Vector analysis of astigmatism changes by flattening, steepening, and torque. *J Cataract Refract Surg.* 1997;23(10):1503-1514.
3. Alpins N, Ong JKY, Stamatelatos G. Asymmetric corneal flattening effect after small incision cataract surgery. *J Refract Surg.* 2016;32(9):598-603.
4. Alpins N, Ong JKY, Stamatelatos G. Refractive surprise after toric intraocular lens implantation: Graph analysis. *J Cataract Refract Surg.* 2014;40(2):283-294.
5. Alpins NA. Wavefront technology: A new advance that fails to answer old questions on corneal vs. refractive astigmatism correction. *J Refract Surg.* 2002;18(6):737-739.
6. Vinas M, Sawides L, de Gracia P, Marcos S. Perceptual adaptation to the correction of natural astigmatism. *PLoS One.* 2012;7(9):e46361.

Chapter 24

Software
ASSORT, iASSORT, Web Calculators, VECTrAK

MANY DIFFERENT PATHS TO SURGICAL SUCCESS

If you don't know where you are going, you'll end up someplace else.
—Yogi Berra

Famed Yankee catcher Yogi Berra's typically off-kilter quip—a misquote of Lewis Carroll—and my own "How do you know how accurate the treatment is if you don't know where the target is," pretty much captures my motivation over the past 30 years: To develop a rational, consistent, scientific framework for mapping a clear pathway to future surgical improvement. I did not want to end up just anywhere; I wanted to end up in a better place and help others do the same. The compendium of my efforts, which were concurrent with the emergence of various techniques and procedures over the years, is contained in the ASSORT (Alpins Statistical System for Ophthalmic Refractive surgery Techniques) Surgical Management System .

The ASSORT Surgical Management System is comprised of 4 separate software programs:

1. **ASSORT**: The flagship total planning and outcomes analysis software designed specifically for ophthalmology with dynamic graphical displays to aid comprehension.

2. **iASSORT**: Designed for topography/tomography and aberrometry devices to calculate the corneal topographic astigmatism (CorT) parameter and use the Alpins Method of vector analysis for change in astigmatism by comparing the numerical parameters on maps over time.

3. **VECTrAK**: A vector calculator that uses the Alpins Method to analyze up to 1000 cases, VECTrAK is capable of importing and exporting data but has no displays.

4. **Web-based calculators**: Freely available at the www.assort.com website, these currently include:
   - Toric Intraocular Lens (IOL) Calculator
   - Femto Limbal Relaxing Incision (LRI) Calculator
   - Vector Planning Calculator
   - Vector Addition and Subtraction Calculator
   - Coupling Calculator

Alpins N. *Practical Astigmatism:*
Planning and Analysis (pp 197-206).
© 2018 SLACK Incorporated.

Figure 24-1. Screen capture from the ASSORT program: Analysis of astigmatic treatment using the Alpins Method. This analysis shows the correction index, angle of error, magnitude of error, and index of success.

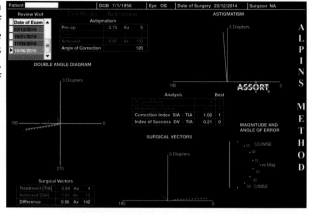

Figure 24-2. Dynamic screen capture from the ASSORT program: Analysis of astigmatism by flattening and torque is shown by the yellow arrows. Flattening is depicted by the yellow arrow pointing to the center of the pupil and torque by the yellow arrow 90° away, producing some rotation in the preoperative astigmatism. The dark green arrow is the SIA and the bright green arrow is the TIA for the incision. The cyan and turquoise rectangles in the center represent the preoperative and postoperative corneal astigmatism respectively. The red dot at the limbus represents the meridian of the incision.

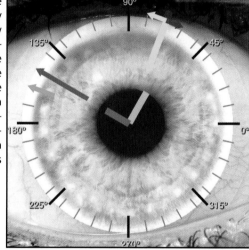

Some of these programs are described elsewhere in this book; the relevant chapters are noted parenthetically below.

THE ASSORT PROGRAM: COMPREHENSIVE APPLICATIONS

The ASSORT program (Figures 24-1 to 24-6) allows for any measurable parameter in ophthalmology to be analyzed and reported. The program uniquely includes the Alpins Method of astigmatism analysis, displayed both numerically and graphically.

Other features of the ASSORT program include:

- Unlimited group reporting on toric IOL, LRI, refractive laser, glaucoma, and other procedures.
- Astigmatism reporting using the targeted induced astigmatism vector (TIA), surgically induced astigmatism vector (SIA), difference vector (DV), correction index (CI), angle of error (AE), magnitude of error (ME), index of success (IOS), coefficient of adjustment (CoA), flattening/steepening of incisions, and torque effect.

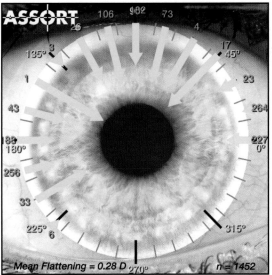

Figure 24-3. Screen capture from the ASSORT program: Analysis of previous phacoemulsification incisions in both the right and left eyes after cataract surgery to determine the amount of flattening. The longer the arrows, the greater the amount of flattening. The numbers around the limbus indicate the number of cases in that 10° sector.

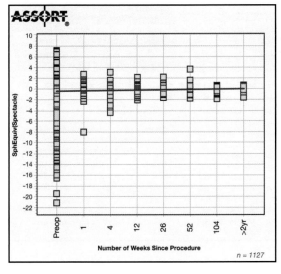

Figure 24-4. Screen capture from the ASSORT program: Scatter graph of spherical equivalent over time post-cataract surgery. Clicking on outlying data points reveals the details of the patient who it represents.

- Surgical vector graphs, bar graphs, and scatter plots as needed.
- Planning of toric IOLs, LRIs, and refractive laser procedures.
- Summated vector means of TIA, SIA, and DV (centroids).

iASSORT FOR CORNEAL TOPOGRAPHER ANALYTICS

The iASSORT program (Chapters 12 and 16) is compatible with most leading topographers/tomographers. iASSORT (Figures 24-7 and 24-8) can be used to calculate CorT anterior and CorT total (incorporating the posterior cornea) from the measured data acquired by the device, which can then be used for planning astigmatic surgery.

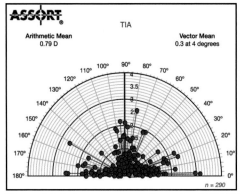

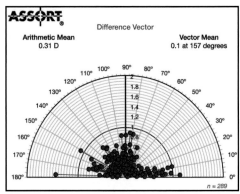

Figure 24-5. Screen capture from the ASSORT program: Surgical vector graph of the TIA displaying the arithmetic mean magnitude of the astigmatism treatments and the summated vector mean.

Figure 24-6. Screen capture from the ASSORT program: Surgical vector graph of the difference vector displaying the arithmetic mean magnitude and the summated vector mean.

Figure 24-7. Screen capture from the iASSORT program: Both CorT anterior and CorT total are calculated. In addition, a corneal astigmatism analysis using the Alpins Method is based here on simulated keratometry (SimK).

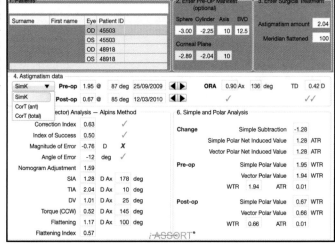

Figure 24-8. Screen capture from the iASSORT program: An astigmatic analysis using a double-angle vector diagram (DAVD) to convert polar to rectangular coordinates.

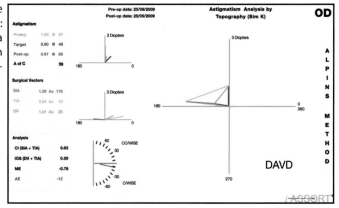

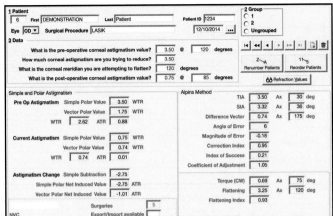

Figure 24-9. Screen capture from the VECTrAK program: The program requires the user to input or import preoperative and postoperative astigmatism parameters. The Alpins Method is used to calculate the surgical success and other outcome elements of the astigmatic correction.

Other features of iASSORT include:
- Graphical and numerical analyses display.
- Analysis of one case at a time using the Alpins Method.
- Calculation of preoperative ocular residual astigmatism (ORA) and topographic disparity (TD).
- Astigmatic analyses using corneal or refractive parameters (second-order refractive cylinder from aberrometry measurements where available).
- Calculation of TIA, SIA, DV, CI, ME, IOS, CoA, and AE.

THE VECTrAK PROGRAM INCLUDES
INTERNAL DATABASE CAPABILITY

The VECTrAK program (Chapters 6, 7, and 8) is a vector calculator, offering a numerical display of Alpins Method astigmatism calculations (Figure 24-9).

The VECTrAK program features the following:
- Allows the import of data (up to 1000 cases) from a spreadsheet and the export of analyses for further statistical processing.
- Allows comparison of up to two groups of interest.

The VECTrAK program does not include a graphical display of the data or analyses.

The Web-based calculators allow analyses of only one case at a time, and have no internal database. These calculations can be complex, so this free, computerized service has been well received for looking at individual patient's results. They are intended to show the user what is available in the ASSORT Surgical Management System where group analyses can then be performed.

Toric Intraocular Lens Calculator

The Toric IOL Calculator (Chapters 10 and 11) offers high accuracy for selecting the most appropriate toric IOL given the preoperative parameters entered (Figures 24-10 through 24-13).

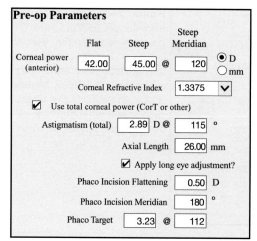

Pre-op Parameters

	Flat	Steep	Steep Meridian	
Corneal power (anterior)	42.00	45.00	@ 120	● D ○ mm

Corneal Refractive Index [1.3375 ▼]

☑ Use total corneal power (CorT or other)

Astigmatism (total) [2.89] D @ [115] °

Axial Length [26.00] mm

☑ Apply long eye adjustment?

Phaco Incision Flattening [0.50] D

Phaco Incision Meridian [180] °

Phaco Target [3.23] @ [112]

Lens type	Sph	Cyl	Expected refraction
HOYA 351T7 Stock	10.50	4.50	0.06 / 0.23 Ax 112
Rayner 573T / 623T Stock	10.50	4.50	-0.10 / 0.16 Ax 112
Medicontur 677TA Stock	10.50	4.50	-0.02 / 0.20Ax 112
ZEISS AT TORBI 709M Stock	11.00	4.50	-0.11 / 0.28 Ax 112
Alsanza Alsiol Toric Stock	10.50	4.50	-0.10 / 0.16 Ax 112
Oculentis LS-313 T5 Stock	10.50	4.50	-0.06 / 0.18 Ax 112
Oculentis LU-313T(Y) Custom	10.41	4.76	0.00 / 0.01 Ax 112
BAUSCH + LOMB MX60T Stock	11.00	5.00	0.01 / 0.01 Ax 112
Mediphacos Miniflex Stock	11.00	5.00	-0.04 / 0.01 Ax 22
Alcon SN60T7 Stock	10.75	4.50	-0.11 / 0.22 Ax 112
Alcon SN6AT7 Stock	11.25	4.50	-0.19 / 0.31 Ax 112
SIFI Medtech V7560CZ Stock	10.50	4.50	0.13 / 0.26 Ax 112
AMO ZCT450 Stock	10.75	4.50	0.05 / 0.29 Ax 112

Figure 24-10. Screen capture from the toric intraocular lens calculator: Numeric input includes options for CorT total, which includes the posterior cornea, and long-eye adjustments.

Figure 24-11. Screen capture from the IOL calculator: Most toric IOLs available worldwide are included in the calculator's selection together with each of their target sphero-cylindrical outcomes.

Figure 24-12. Screen capture from the ASSORT dynamic IOL calculator: The expected refraction for most of the toric IOLs available worldwide is calculated based on the preoperative parameters entered.

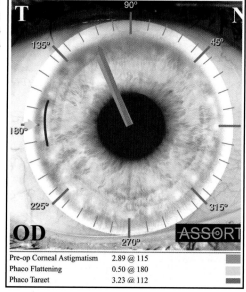

Pre-op Corneal Astigmatism	2.89 @ 115
Phaco Flattening	0.50 @ 180
Phaco Target	3.23 @ 112

Features of the toric IOL calculator include:
- Employing CorT total using measurements of the posterior cornea for an accurate astigmatic value.
- The specifications of most toric IOLs available worldwide are programmed into the calculator.
- Displaying the expected spherocylinder for all appropriate toric IOLs.
- IOL constants can be personalized using the SRK/T, Holladay 1, Hoffer Q, or Haigis formulas.[1-4]

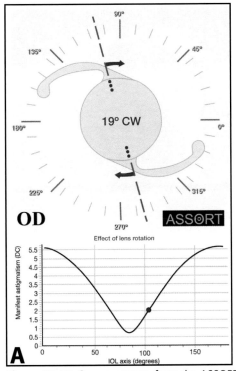

Alpins Method

SIA	3.48	Ax	42
TIA	2.90	Ax	25
Difference Vector	1.94	Ax	160
Correction Index	1.20		
Index of Success	0.67		
Magnitude of Error	0.59		
B　Angle of Error	17 (CCW)		

Figure 24-13. Screen capture from the ASSORT IOL program: (A) Postoperative toric IOL analysis allows the user to determine if the implanted IOL can be rotated to improve for any refractive cylinder surprise. (B) A vector analysis for each individual eye is provided to quantify the ME for toric implant power.

- Wang-Koch adjustment for long eyes can be calculated.
- Calculations are transparent to the user.
- The calculator offers postoperative vectorial analyses to solve refractive surprises, including graphical and numerical displays of expected manifest refraction after rotation of the IOL.

Femto Limbal Relaxing Incision Calculator

The Femto LRI Calculator (Chapters 8 and 12) performs a vectorial calculation of the effect of the phacoemulsification incision and the limbal relaxing incision on the preoperative corneal astigmatism and its correction (Figure 24-14).

The Femto LRI Calculator offers:
- Use of 7 LRI nomograms, including Nichamin and Donnenfeld nomograms[5]
- Display of polar and double-angle vector diagrams (DAVDs)
- Graphical display of LRI incision magnitude and location
- Performs a vectorial analysis for outcomes and nomogram calculation

Figure 24-14. Screen capture from the femto LRI calculator: The graphical display shows the planned incisions on the eye after selecting a listed nomogram.

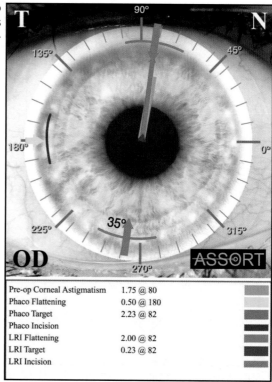

Pre-op Corneal Astigmatism	1.75 @ 80
Phaco Flattening	0.50 @ 180
Phaco Target	2.23 @ 82
Phaco Incision	
LRI Flattening	2.00 @ 82
LRI Target	0.23 @ 82
LRI Incision	

Vector Planning Calculator

The Vector Planning Calculator (Chapters 13 and 14) is used for refractive excimer laser treatments (Figure 24-15).

The Vector Planning Calculator offers:

- Calculation of ORA using manifest refraction, wavefront refraction, or cycloplegic refraction compared with corneal topography, keratometry, or CorT.
- Incorporating corneal astigmatism into astigmatic treatment plan (TIA) using 99 different emphasis points.
- Target spherical equivalent can be set by user.
- Mixed astigmatism treatments using planocylindrical ablations can be calculated.
- Surgical vectors including the TIA at all 99 emphasis points can be displayed.
- Target corneal astigmatism and refractive cylinder are calculated to determine

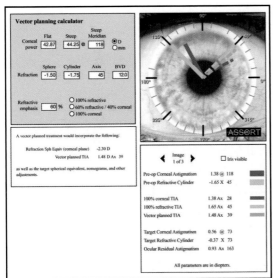

Figure 24-15. Screen capture from the Vector Planning Calculator: The Vector Planning Calculator incorporates the corneal and refractive cylinder parameters into the treatment plan for refractive excimer laser procedures. This facility reduces corneal and refractive astigmatism.

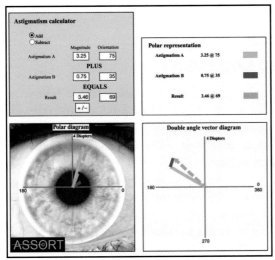

Figure 24-16. Screen capture from the Vector Planning Calculator: The Vector Planning Calculator incorporates the corneal and refractive cylinder parameters into the treatment plan for refractive excimer laser procedures. This facility reduces corneal and refractive astigmatism.

Vector Calculator

The Vector Calculator (Chapters 2, 5, 6, and 7) calculates addition or subtraction of any two astigmatisms (refractive and/or corneal) (Figure 24-16).

The Vector Calculator:
- Offers graphical display of vectors including DAVDs and how they appear on an eye.
- Can be calculated in plus or minus cylinder form.

Coupling Calculator

The Coupling Calculator (Chapter 21) calculates the change in the spherical component of any treatment as a result of the astigmatic treatment for both incisional (cataract)

Figure 24-17. Screen capture from the Coupling Calculator: Displays the coupling ratio, coupling adjustment, and the new clinically significant coupling adjustment for any effect of the astigmatism treatment on the spherical component of the treatment.

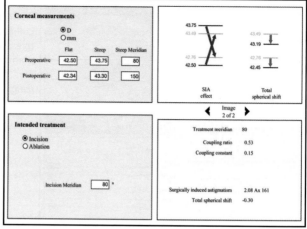

and ablative (excimer laser) procedures (Figure 24-17). Diagrams display step-by-step calculation of the coupling ratio, coupling constant, and coupling adjustment. Off-axis and under/over correction effects are taken into account.

Service to Colleagues

I appreciate the opportunity to provide this information about the offerings of ASSORT Pty. Ltd, of Melbourne, Australia, which provides these products and services. I have an obvious financial interest in the material, but ASSORT has always extended maximum attention and responsiveness to queries from colleagues and customers. We also offer as much as we can for free on the website.

This book has also given me the chance, through copious referencing, to honor the hundreds of centers and individuals around the world who have contributed to this area of ophthalmic endeavor. My contributions are but one corner of this world, and it is simply not possible to fully express my appreciation to those who have helped me and my team over the years.

References

1. Retzlaff JA, Sanders DR, Kraff MC. Development of the SRK/T intraocular lens implant power calculation formula. *J Cataract Refract Surg.* 1990;16(3):333-340.
2. Holladay JT, Prager TC, Chandler TY, Musgrove KH, Lewis JW, Ruiz RS. A three-part system for refining intraocular lens power calculations. *J Cataract Refract Surg.* 1988;14(1):17-24.
3. Hoffer KJ. The Hoffer Q formula: a comparison of theoretic and regression formulas. *J Cataract Refract Surg.* 1993;19(6):700-712.
4. Haigis W. The Haigis Formula. In: Shammas HJ, ed. *Intraocular Lens Power Calculations.* Thorofare, NJ: SLACK Incorporated; 2004:41-47.
5. Holladay JT. Standardizing constants for ultrasonic biometry, keratometry, and intraocular lens power calculations. *J Cataract Refract Surg.* 1997;23(9):1356-1370.

Appendix
Astigmatic Terms and Concepts

1. Corneal astigmatism and vectors should always be displayed as positive; to convert from negative astigmatism to positive astigmatism, change the polar meridian by 90°.

2. When referring to corneal astigmatism, the orientation of the astigmatism should be referred to as "meridian." When referring to corneal refractive cylinder correction, the direction should be referred to as "axis," which for a negative cylinder is 90° away.

3. Use the @ symbol for corneal astigmatism and "X" for refractive cylinder.

4. All refractive cylinder parameters should be converted to the corneal plane before analyzing astigmatic outcomes.

5. The effect of corneal incisions on corneal astigmatism should be quantified using the flattening effect (FE), not the surgically induced astigmatism vector (SIA), as it is the FE that determines the amount of flattening separately from the rotation or torque at the incision meridian. The SIA parameter is the total astigmatic change and incorporates both the flattening or steepening effect and the torque.

6. It is the FE that is the required input in toric intraocular lens (IOL) calculators to determine the amount of corneal astigmatism that is to be neutralized by the toric IOL and not the whole SIA.

7. Astigmatic analyses in refractive surgery should be performed using both refractive and corneal parameters. Remember, there is only one common target induced astigmatism vector (TIA) for both analyses.

Alpins N. *Practical Astigmatism:
Planning and Analysis* (pp 207-208).
© 2018 SLACK Incorporated.

8. Polar diagrams, which are usually on a 180° fan display, can also be displayed on a 360° diagram to show the superior topography separately from the inferior topography and the separate hemidivisional vectorial change.

9. A double-angle display taking astigmatisms from 180° to 360° for the purposes of statistical analysis of preoperative and postoperative astigmatism values is not a vectorial analysis of change. It is just a display of astigmatisms at twice their existing meridian.

10. The toric IOL 10-point check table can be used to determine what various calculators are including or missing from their calculations (see Chapter 10). This will change as calculators are upgraded by the respective companies.

11. Vector analysis shows that a toric IOL misalignment of 15° reduces the astigmatic correction effect by 13.6%, not 50% as is incorrectly cited by many. This latter value is a scalar analysis of change by comparing postoperative cylinder and preoperative astigmatisms.

12. Scalar comparisons of postoperative and preoperative astigmatism give limited information about where the process in astigmatism correction was inaccurate. To understand the process, a vectorial analysis is required.

13. The maximum ablation in refractive laser surgery occurs at the negative refractive cylinder axis (tissue removal), whereas corneal incisions to reduce astigmatism are placed on the steep corneal meridian (net tissue addition).

14. Ocular residual astigmatism (ORA) refers to the vectorial difference between corneal astigmatism and the refractive cylinder at the corneal plane encompassing the whole visual pathway to the cerebral cortex. It should not be confused with residual astigmatism, postoperative astigmatism, lenticular astigmatism, or internal astigmatism.

15. Postoperative astigmatism present after the completion of surgery should preferably be referred to as "remaining" or "resultant" astigmatism. Use of the commonly employed term residual astigmatism is easily confused with ocular residual astigmatism, which Duke Elder described as "residual astigmatism."

Financial Disclosures

Dr. Noel Alpins is CEO of ASSORT Surgical Management Systems.

Dr. Dan Z. Reinstein is a consultant for Carl Zeiss Meditec and has financial interest in ArcScan, Inc.

Dr. Spencer P. Thornton has not disclosed any relevant financial relationships.

Index